To Nurse Means to Nurture

The Need for Nurses to Comfort their Patients

Preface

This is a much needed book to help educate nurses to how profoundly their behavior affects sensitive patients, like my sweet dear autistic husband, who are in their care. Because there is a shortage of nurses they are not held accountable for how they treat patients who in turn makes the lives of people who deal with the patient when they go home extremely difficult. They don't see the aftermath. Brian has written an amazing book straight from his heart. He has spent many precious hours looking through magazines and reading through tons of medical books in order to find what he calls "proof" that bringing their patients comfort is indeed an important part of a nurse's job. He was careful to tell you in great detail where he found each piece of information so you wouldn't think he made it up. A great portion of the information came from a college textbook, Fundamentals of Nursing or the actual exam that nurses have to pass in order to become a nurse. I believe if nurses knew what a huge impact they had on their patients lives there would be nurse reform.

Bertha Marie Evans

Introduction

In this book you will find quotes from encyclopedias both old and new as well as some of my past medical assisting books, dictionaries both old and new defining words, as well as other health books and other books pertaining to the medical field regarding the fact that nurses are supposed to comfort their patients. I even found a college textbook of nursing that was on sale at the Library I just recently bought so I could use some of the comments I could find in it about comforting your patients in nursing care, and I found several. They were all over the place. You will be surprised and you will be shocked at what you will find when you read my book concerning what all these different sources had to say about nurses comforting their patients, including several from the college book of nursing. The college book I bought at a Library Book Sale was "Fundamentals of Nursing, 7th Edition, 2009." These quotes are all over their book and yes that includes touching your patients not just standing back and putting on a smile. This came with a CD that had Videos matching the chapters, but the CD was not included when it was donated to the library by a nursing student so I was unable to see these videos. I did however get to see nurses in action from the DVD "Facing Death" 2009, and, "Nursing-Care Career Book and DVD, 2008" and they showed the nurses in action actually comforting their patients in the exact same manner as I am asking you to comfort me. And, the patients on the DVD that came with the Nursing-Care Career Book and DVD that were being comforted by their nurses in various ways were my age, and were not dying. They were just having procedures done. Also, if you run into a place where I'm actually doing all the talking for 3 or 4 pages, probably in the last half of the book, don't stop reading, there's more quotes to come. You're not to the end of the quotes yet. They're all throughout the book all the way to the end. You will also encounter examples of how nurses have comforted their patients found in kid books about nursing, adult DVDs about nursing, and a few adult books about nursing. In some instances you will even see actual comments made by others about how nurses comforted them or someone else.

Believe it or not, I have actually spotted comments in books and articles such as "my doctor put their arm around me" or "and the nurse stroked their face", or, "and Clara Barton cradled him in her arms" (a nurse holding a soldier in her arms). I've even seen nurses in action on modern day DVDs about nursing rubbing their patients' head, holding their hand, and stroking their face. What I am getting at is some nurses say it is not in their job description to comfort their patients, especially in this manner, when in fact, I have the proof that it is in their job description, even on their nurse exam, and I have proof that nurses do comfort their patients in the exact manner I'm asking them to comfort me in this very book. Be prepared to read my book and see for yourself the enlightening truth.

Synopsis
To Nurse Means to Nurture

To Nurse means to nurture. Nurture in the dictionary also means nourish. I like a spelling thesaurus gadget a friend gave me. I don't really have trouble spelling. I just play with it for kicks to get meanings of words. According to this thesaurus gadget a friend at bingo gave me, the word nurse means "to act as a parent to." I've been looking for this definition the whole time. That's what I thought it meant.

To those who wish to be nurses, you are not just taking on a profession where you stick patients with a bunch of needles and help with surgeries and then receive a paycheck for it. You are acting as a parent to these people. You are their caretaker and you are actually supposed to treat these people that are your patients like they are your children while they are under your care. Anything you would do for your child from a comforting standpoint needs to be done for your patients. That's why I believe one of the people I copied the quote of in my book said that being a nurse is a great teaching tool for how to raise your kids. I think they meant that you were supposed to comfort them and console them in their fear and pain with great compassion. And, they did say in their quote that you are supposed to comfort your patients, by the way. That means if they need you to pat them on the shoulder, or give them a hug, or rub their head to calm them down and hold their hand you need to do so. You would do this for your kids wouldn't you? Your patients need you to do the same for them no matter what their age. In case you think I am the only one emphasizing age, one of the people I quoted said that comfort should not be left to end of life care but that people of all ages should be comforted by their nurses. So, please remember to reevaluate your responsibility as a nurse and remember that comforting your patients is the key to good patient care. By the way, one of your own medical professionals also made this quote almost exactly. I'm just confirming it. You didn't know I knew all this did you? Please make sure to remember to comfort me and all your patients when they come your way. Thank you.

To Nurse Means To Nurture
The Need for Nurses to Comfort their Patients

My name is Brian Evans and I am autistic and have a need to receive a lot of affection from those around me because of my disability, especially because of a lot of the sensory issues I have that make me need the childlike needs I have. Believe it or not, I actually know a little bit about medical terminology and a little bit about how the environment of the nursing world is supposed to work. Some nurses think it is just to give shots and blood tests and just stand back and smile while the patient is suffering in pain and not comfort them at all when this is what they need because they think this is all they are required to do and are only there for the paycheck. I want to plead with you to listen to what I have to say because I have taken some classes myself in your field of study but I was going for office work rather than clinical work and heard things from teachers and read things in books that might surprise you. The Director of the Medical Assisting Program I took classes in actually got up in front of her class and told her students, "If a patient comes to you and asks you to comfort them a certain way, you have to do it. If a patient comes to you and asks for a certain person they are comfortable with, or asks for a female instead of a male, or asks for a specific person they are comfortable with to work with them, you have to give it to them. It's not about the nurse's rights. It's the patient's rights that matter. It doesn't matter how you feel or what you want to do, if a patient asks you to do certain things for them to comfort them through a needle stick you have to do it." I even read a page in one of the college textbooks she gave us that said the exact same thing. I would like to share with you a few important facts about the bedside manner of nurses that are needed that seem to not be known to those in the nursing world. Just because you are nice and do a good job does not make you a good nurse alone, you need to be willing to go out of your way to meet the emotional needs of your patient and be willing to comfort your patients when they come to you for you to take care of them. They're not coming to you to do business with you. They are coming to you for you to "take care of them". A parent "takes care of" their child. A nursing home "takes care of" its residents. A hospital "takes care of" its patients.

A doctor's office "takes care of" its patients. You, as a nurse "take care of" your patients. Did you realize what that means? Have you ever heard the phrase "tender loving care" often used to describe a particularly compassionate nurse or doctor? I would like to define for you what some words mean that are commonly used in nursing that describe good nursing practice that pleases people to help nurses understand what these words really mean. Here is what these words mean.

If you take the words "tender loving care" and dissect them, this is what this means.

Tender – kind, affectionate, gentle
Loving- affectionate; devoted, kind
Care- to have or show regard, interest; to look after or provide for; to feel interest concerning: also to have a fondness or like

> Funk & Wagnall's Standard Desk Dictionary Volume 1 A-M, page 94, 1984
> Funk & Wagnall's Standard Desk Dictionary Volume 1 A-M, page 384, 1984
> Funk & Wagnall's Standard Desk Dictionary Volume 2 N-Z, page 696, 1984

So, showing tender loving care would mean to be devoted to your work by showing interest in your patients by providing kindness, gentleness and affection and show concern for how your patient feels. Bring them the comfort they need. What do they need you to do to comfort them? Do this for them if you want to show tender loving care because that's what tender loving care is, showing kindness, gentleness, and affection.

Tender is a kind, loving, solicitous; feeling, expressing, affection.

Tender is also soft hearted; easily touched; sympathetic, a tender feeling person; kind, compassionate of, pitiful; affectionate or loving, sentimental or amatory, considerate or careful, sensitive.
The American College Dictionary, page 1247, 1959

Have you ever heard the phrase "compassionate care"?

Let me break this down for you as well.

Compassionate- feeling compassion or pity, merciful, sympathetic.

Compassion is pity for the suffering or the distress of another with the desire to help or spare.

Care- to have or show regard, interest; to look after or provide for; to feel interest concerning: also to have a fondness or like; to desire, to want

>Funk & Wagnall's Standard Desk Dictionary Volume 1, A-M, page 128, 1984
>Funk & Wagnall's Standard Desk Dictionary Volume 1, A-M, page 94, 1984

So, you see, to have compassionate care you need to have pity for the suffering or distress of your patients and show interest in their needs and provide for the needs they have and comfort them the way they need to be comforted, not how you decide you want to comfort them, but how they need you to comfort them.

You also have the desire to show mercy to your patients and want to help them when you show them compassionate care.

What comforts them? Find out what comforts them and meet their requests for comfort. If they need hugs, give them hugs. If they need a pat on the shoulder, give them a pat. If they need their head rubbed, rub their head. If they need their hand held, hold their hand. Treat them as if they were one of your own children and treat them like a child and provide comfort for them in the way you would provide comfort for a child. And, don't give me this "High 5s" bit and say that's how you do it because I know better than that. You know very well you're not going to give a scared child who comes to you for comfort in their distress High 5's. That would have been considered "horseplay" by my 2nd and 3rd grade teachers, "not comfort".

And this "shaking hands" bit isn't comfort, either. I don't even understand why some people even consider that a greeting. The public doesn't understand that "handshakes were never originally meant for greeting people" as they think. "Handshakes were used to 'break deals' on 'business propositions'", "not greet people". I even found out reading some historical account that Thomas Jefferson or whoever the president was in 1801 only introduced handshakes in congress "in order to get out of having to bow to kings" because it was less straining to do that than to bow. You see, he wasn't doing that to greet the every day person; he was doing that as an alternative way to greet royalty with honor when he was really supposed to "bow". This isn't the way you comfort a child or anybody else. There's nothing comforting about it. Neither is this new thing I recently found out you came up with called "bumping arms". I never even heard of such a thing until recently. I don't understand what's got into everybody. Not only that my 2nd and 3rd grade teachers would have also considered that as being "horseplay" as well. No one comforts their child like this. I've never seen a parent or teacher or nurse comfort a child that way. You know good and well you would give them a hug, pat their shoulder, rub their head, maybe even rub their shoulder, or hold their hand, or all the above. This is how parents and teachers and nurses always comforted children, by giving them hugs, shoulder pats, head rubs, and shoulder rubs, and holding their hand. You do this for them all the time. This other gibberish people are coming up with about handshakes, high 5's and bumping arms is ridiculous. You give your kids hugs, shoulder pats, head rubs, and shoulder rubs and hand holds all the time. You need to do this for your patients all the time as well. How have you seen nurses show comfort to their nursing home residents?

I tell you what I've seen. I've seen them comfort them the very same way I am asking you to comfort me, so technically, the ways I'm asking you to comfort me are not out of line as some nurses would think.

I'm just asking you to comfort me the way you would comfort your own children and the way nursing home nurses would comfort their senior citizens residents.

This is what I need and I want to be able to show you how I know you are supposed to meet these needs. Please bear with me and let me speak my peace. I wish to help you understand.

I just recently found the following section on "Love Needs in Illness" from Basic Nursing: A Psychophysiologic Approach, Sorensen Luckman, 1979, W.B. Saunders Company to help prove my point about the way nurses are supposed to comfort their patients. This is kind of long, so bear with me, what you're supposed to do is in the very last paragraph of this section. Here goes:

"Separation from one's usual companions and way of life means that needs for love, belonging, and closeness are severely threatened in the existence of the ill. We are referring not only to romantic or physical love but also to those strong feelings of "affection", "concern", "kindness", "closeness", and "understanding" that one shares with significant others close to him. These shared feelings are essential for a feeling of well – being; and therefore, their absence creates a most unhappy situation. When ill and away from those persons they care about, patients obviously worry: "Will loved ones change" Will they no longer want me? Am I an unattractive burden?"

> Basic Nursing: A Psychophysiologic Approach, Sorenson, Luckman, 1979, W. B. Saunders Company, page 159

"Like the stimulation needs and the needs for safety and security, the needs for "love" and "belonging" are present in "all patients". These "important needs" are "not vaporized by illness". In fact, they "may be intensified by the uncertainty of the illness and by illness itself". As we mentioned, the persons who provide gratification of needs "may shift somewhat with the illness": when he was well, the patient's needs were gratified by individuals in his private life; with illness he now looks to those in the "health care professions" for "need gratification".

> Basic Nursing: A Psychophysiologic Approach, Sorenson, Luckman, 1979, W. B. Saunders Company, page 159

"We do not mean to imply that staff members can ever take the place of friends and relatives for the patient; nor do we mean to imply that loved ones cease to provide need gratification to contribute to the ever-present needs for safety, security, "love" and belonging that continue into a patient's existence in a care facility.

> Basic Nursing: A Psychophysiologic Approach, Sorenson, Luckman, 1979, W. B. Saunders Company, page 159

In these settings staff members "may be with a patient more than loved ones are", also they are often with him during "crisis moments" in his life and illness when loved ones may be excluded from his presence, e.g., surgery, intensive care, isolation and emergencies."

> Basic Nursing: A Psychophysiologic Approach, Sorenson, Luckman, 1979, W. B. Saunders Company, page 159

"Patients worry about 'being treated impersonally'. A "touch of the hand", "a stroke on the brow", "a look", "and a pat", "the way a patient is handled", "made comfortable", and "helped" can all contribute to making him feel valued and "close" to "those caring for him". In all these "loving-caring gestures" the nurse remembers that her actions should not be seductive in nature but rather are in sincere expression of appropriate concern."

> Basic Nursing: A Psychophysiologic Approach, Sorenson, Luckman, 1979, W. B. Saunders Company, page 159

A patient is not truly "taken care of" unless "the nurse" helps him to feel "safe", "secure', "loved", and as one who "belongs" rather than as an outsider who is viewed as an intruder."

> Basic Nursing: A Psychophysiologic Approach, Sorenson, Luckman, 1979, W. B. Saunders Company, page 159

In my particular situation, I do not feel safe unless "the nurse" is the one doing the "comforting", and the nurse is a "cheery acting" nurse. All of them need to be "cheery acting" and all of them need to be "females" and all of them need to "give me hugs" and "rub my head to calm me down and hold my hand through needle sticks". If someone who is with me tries to do the comforting it feels like it is me and them against the nurse.

If a nurse does the comforting, "a chipper acting, cheery female nurse" while another "chipper acting cheery female nurse does the needle sticks" I feel like I am being loved and protected by those taking care of me, "the nurses" when they do this for me and it makes me feel at peace with my nurses when they do this for me.

I still need to let you know, though, that I'll probably still scream and cry through the needle sticks when you stick me because I have a severe oversensitivity to pain, but I will feel safer with the people sticking me if they are the ones I am comfortable with and they do what I need them to do that comforts me.

"Male doctors", "male nurses" and "serious trended female nurses" "tortured me as a child" and "serious trended female nurses" continued to "torture me throughout my adulthood".

The "cheery acting ones" are always good with me and they are the only ones I am comfortable with.

My nurses have to be the "chipper acting, cheery female nurses or it's not going to work. No one else will do.

Nurses should have mercy on their patients in the fear and pain and show sympathy to them and comfort them in their fear and pain.

Let me define mercy and sympathy for you and work up to comfort to show you what these really mean.

Mercy- A disposition to be kind, forgiving, or helpful; mercy comes from compassion, kindness, or other ennobling sentiment
> Funk & Wagnall's Standard Desk Dictionary, Volume 1, A-M, page 407, 1984

Merciful means full of or exercising mercy.
> Funk & Wagnall's Standard Desk Dictionary, Volume 1, A-M, page 406, 1984

Spare- To free or relieve someone from pain or to be lenient or forgiving.
> Funk & Wagnall's Standard Desk Dictionary, Volume 2,
> N-Z, page 645, 1984

Sympathy–The quality of being affected by the state of another with feeling correspondent in kind. 2. A fellow feeling; especially a feeling of compassion for another's suffering; pity; commiseration 3. An agreement of "affections", inclinations, or temperaments that make persons agreeable to one another; congenially
> Funk & Wagnall's Standard Desk Dictionary, Volume 2,
> N-Z, page 645, 1984

Congenially – Having similar character or tastes; sympathetic 2. Suited to one's disposition; agreeable
> Funk & Wagnall's Standard Desk Dictionary, Volume 1,
> A-M, page 134, 1984

Disposition- One's usual frame of mind; temperament
> Funk & Wagnall's Standard Desk Dictionary, Volume 1,
> A-M, page 185, 1984

So sympathy in medical care would be showing compassion for a patient's suffering by agreement of affections that are suited to the patient's disposition, which fit their usual frame of mind. So, if they need a hug, you give them a hug. If they need a pat on the shoulder, you give them a pat on the shoulder. If they need you to rub their head to comfort them, you rub their head. If they need you to hold their hand, you need to hold their hand to comfort them the way they need comforted and not the way you decide you want to comfort them.

When a patient asks you for comfort and they need you to comfort them the way you would a child, don't think of it as "This stranger over here wants to get intimate with me. What's the deal with them?" Think of it as "This poor soul that came in here today to receive my care needs me to give them a hug or pat them on the shoulder or rub their head or hold their hand because their scared when they have to see the doctor and shots and blood tests and IVs hurt and I need to comfort this poor person." When you think of it this way, you are thinking of it in the correct context because this is exactly what is taking place here. Your patients do not come to you as a stranger just looking for special attention, they are coming to you as a person in need that needs you to doctor them up and comfort them in their distress and be reassured you are their friend and you will do what you can to help them and be treated by you as if they were one of your own children.

A senior citizen came to me at Bingo one day and gave me this spelling thesaurus electronic gadget that gave definitions to what words mean you type in there. Take a wild guess what came up when I typed the word "nurse" in there, "to act as a parent to."

If you look "nurse" up in the dictionary it will also tell you "nurse" means to "nurture".

I bet that's a shock isn't it.

So, now maybe you won't be so shocked when you see what the definition of comfort is.

Comfort- to soothe when in grief; console; cheer 2. To make "physically" comfortable 3. To aid; encourage 4. Relief in affliction; consolation, solace 5. The feeling of relief or consolation 6. A person or thing that affords consolation 7. A cause or matter or relief or satisfaction 8. a "satisfaction of bodily wants" 9. That which promotes strengthening aid; assistance 10. A comforter, bed cover 11. Comforter
      The American College Dictionary, page 241, Random
      House Incorporated, 1959

Provide – to supply or furnish
> The American College Dictionary, page 975, Random
> House Incorporated, 1959

To provide comfort would be to supply comfort. To provide
tender loving care would be to supply kind, gentle, affection out of
concern for the patient and what they need.

Here are some more definitions of what tender means.
Tender- affectionate or loving
> American College Dictionary, page 1247, Random House
> Incorporated, 1959

Tender – kind, loving, solicitous; feeling, "expressing affection", a
tender glance, "touch", tender care; careful not to wound;
considerate: be tender of his conscientious scruples, tender of
hurting his feelings
> Webster's Universal Dictionary, page 1538, Routledge &
> Keagan Paul LTD., 1968

Tenderness- 1. Delicacy, softness of texture 2. Sensitiveness to
pain 3. Sensitive to the suffering of others; compassionateness,
tenderness of heart; moral scruple; tenderness of conscience 4.
"Affection", "love", solicitude; "expression of these in action and
behavior' kindness, gentleness.
> Webster's Universal Dictionary, page 1538, Routledge &
> Kegan Paul LTD., 1968

Here's the definition of what a tenderhearted person is.

Tenderhearted – having a tender heart; susceptible; easily moved
by; pity, kind, compassionate
> Webster's Universal Dictionary, page 1538, Routledge &
> Kegan Paul LTD., 1968

Sometimes Bertha will tell someone they need to caress the top of
my head to calm me down through a needle stick which would be
the same as rubbing my head to calm me down.

Believe it or not this is one thing some nurses do for their patients, and even though they may not do this for everybody, some have done the same for a few others that were either ill or scared or in pain because this is something nurses do to help their patients when they see them.

Here is the definition of Caress.

Caress – an act or gesture expressing affection as an embrace, pat; to touch in affection, to treat with favor, kindness, etc.
> Funk & Wagnall's Standard Dictionary, A-M, page 94, 1985

A caretaker is the one who does this for their patients. This would be their nurse. Here is the definition of a caretaker.

Caretaker- a person who takes care of a person, place, or thing
> Funk & Wagnall's Standard Dictionary, A-M, page 94, 1985

Here are some other words for nurse I found in a very old thesaurus.

Nurse means cherish, foster tend, feed, encourage, nurture, nourish, "pamper".
> A Dictionary of Synonyms & Antonyms, Warner Books Edition, 1938 & 1961

Pamper- to treat very indulgently; gratify the whims or "wishes of"; "coddle"
> Funk & Wagnall's Standard Dictionary, Volume 1, A-M, ` page 471, 1985

Coddle – "to treat as a baby" or an invalid; "pamper"
> Funk & Wagnall's Standard Dictionary, Volume 1, A-M, page 121, 1985

Does this shock you? Yes, nurses are supposed to pamper their patients when they come to them especially when being seen for a procedure to help comfort them through their pain and anxiety.

There have been some nurses recently that told me that "physical contact" was not part of their requirement to meet their patients' emotional needs. Where some understand my need for affection, others think it out of line for me to want to touch them or ask them to touch me.

To clarify that meeting the emotional needs of your patients does include "physical contact" including "touch" I'd like you to read the following nurses' creed by M.A. Haggerty that some nurses may have missed reading in their training, and I believe Florence Nightingale would have told you the same thing as well.

Here is the Nurses' Creed I found

The Nurses Creed by M.A. Haggerty, RN says, "Lord, let me begin today with your blessing to provide care for those who need me. Give me the patience to listen, intuition to see beyond the visible, knowledge to practice the art of nursing, and the attitude to deliver care with humility. Help me to see every patient clearly unbiased, and with individual respect help me to face fear and anxiety with kind words and a gentle touch. Help me to see the joy and wonder each new day brings. And let your healing light shine through my hands."

Did you notice something interesting about this quote? It says, "Help me to see every patient clearly unbiased, and with individual respect help me to face fear and anxiety with "kind words" and "a gentle touch".

Notice anything else about this quote. It also says, "And let your healing light 'shine through my hands'."

There have been some nurses in my recent past that said it was not in their list of requirements to "comfort their patients".

Others have been very receptive to the idea and have given right in and did well with me but the ones that said they thought that wasn't in their job description seemed unwilling to budge an inch to hug me or comfort me either one because they thought it was improper or out of line.

Actually, think again, there really are things in the medical field confirming that nurses do in fact need to comfort their patients. I have several quotes that verify this very fact.

Here are some resources that verify the fact that nurses are supposed to comfort their patients in the hospital setting. Please read the following quotes and see for yourself that there really are indicators in the field of medicine that nurses are required to comfort their patients. I have several pages of references here that say that very thing.

According to Glencoe Health a Certified Surgical Technologist (CST) will demonstrate the following upon completion of an approved program:

1. Knowledge of surgical aseptic (cleansing) techniques;

2. Familiarity with basic surgical procedures, with anatomy, physiology, and microbiology, and with pathological processes;

3. The ability to meet patient's need for comfort, safety, and reassurance;

4. The ability to anticipate and meet the needs of the surgical team and function in areas where qualified.

Notice this says, "Ability to meet the patient's comfort" in number 3. It also says to meet their need for "reassurance".

This book directs its nurses to the American Medical Association's Committee on Allied Health Education and Accreditation, or the Association of Surgical Technologists.

This is on page 265 of the Glenco Health textbook for Health students.

Also, according to Glenco Health, LPNs and LVNs perform many of the patient-care duties, teaching them good health practices, assisting with rehabilitation, and offering comfort and emotional reassurance during times of suffering and crisis.

Notice it says "Perform Patient duties", one of which is to "Comfort" their patients and give them "emotional reassurance".
This is on page 441 of the Glenco Health textbook for Health Students.
Glenco, McGraw-Hill, 19

CODE OF ETHICS for the Medical Assistant:

"The Code of Ethics of this Association shall set forth principles of ethical and moral conduct as they relate to the medical profession and the particular practice of medical assisting. Members of this Association dedicated to the conscientious pursuit of their profession, and thus desiring to merit the high regard of the entire medical profession and the respect of the general public which they serve, do pledge themselves to strive always to render service to humanity with full respect for the dignity of each person; respect confidential information gained through employment unless legally authorized or required by responsible performance of duty to divulge such information; uphold the honor and high principles of the profession and accept its disciplines; seek to continually improve our knowledge and skills of medical assisting for the benefit of patients and professional colleagues; and participate in additional service activities which aim toward improving the health and well-being for the community."
The Administrative Medical Assistant, Mary E. Kein, 1988, 2nd Edition, page36.

Notice this not only says they are to aim toward improving the health of the community but also the "well-being" of the community and comforting your patients in your care helps to improve their "well-being".

"Much of what you do as a nurse is based on sympathy, empathy, compassion and your want to care."

>How to Books –Working as a Nurse, Esther Bartlett and Marion Field, 1999, page 32

The Florence Nightingale Pledge goes like this, "I solemnly pledge myself before God and in the presence of this assembly, to pass my life in purity and to practice my profession faithfully. I will abstain from whatever is deleterious and mischievous, and will not take or knowingly administer any harmful drug. I will do all in my power to maintain and elevate the standard of my profession, and will hold in confidence all personal matters committed to my keeping and all family affairs coming to my knowledge in the practice of my calling. With loyalty will I endeavor to aid the physician in his work, and devote myself to the welfare of those committed to my care."

>American Nurses Association
>The Nightingale Tribute (Kansas State Nurses Association website)

Notice she said she wanted to devote herself to the "welfare" of those committed to her care.

Welfare in this instance would probably pass for the definition of "faring well" or "aiding those in need".

Here are even more quotes in regards to nurses comforting their patients.

Comfort: Nurse's First and Last Consideration
"Nowadays, you can see nurses in hospitals receiving a number of patients. Unaware of their actions during initial interaction comfort has been forgotten and out of priority."

>By Grepaz Isaac, RN, Quezon City, Philippines

"While a lot is written about the bullying that can go on within the nursing profession, Christine Szweda RN, BSN, MS, NE-BC, director of nursing education for competency and assessment at the Cleveland Clinic believes nurses can instead provide each other with a powerful support network."

> Nursezone.com
> For Work for Life

"When it comes to patient care, nurses consistently play the role or advocate as they support each patient's emotional well-being, contribute to the healing process and speak on their patient's behalf. Nurses can also put their advocacy skills to work in advocating for each other and for the profession as a whole"

> Meagan M. Krishka, contributor, Nursezone.com
> For Work or For Life

"Everyone is capable of showing care and giving comfort…whether it is for someone so close to you or even for a bystander needing help or assistance…Giving comfort or showing care is not stated in books, it comes out naturally… They say you cannot be a nurse when you don't know how to care and you don't care at all…I definitely agree to that… A nurse is always judged by her ability to make her patients comfortable. As nurses, we are the comfort providers…we don't simply follow doctor's orders and give medications in an instant, instead, we dig deeper…we empathize…we do our own interventions within our scope of responsibility giving emphasis on provided simple comfort measures."

> By Dianne Kristin G. Pella., R.N.
> Calcoon City, Philippines
> Sunday, July 11, 2010
> A Novice Nurse

Notice this quote above says "As nurses, we are the comfort providers".

It says nurses not only follow doctor's orders and hand out medications but they do their interventions within their scope of responsibility to provide simple "comfort measures".

The Director of my Medical Assisting Program I took classes in also got up in front of class one day and told her students that in the case of a mother and child, when it comes to nurses dealing with the patient and comforting the patient, it is usually best to let the nurse be the ones to deal with the patient and comfort them themselves.

 It usually works out better when the child being comforted is able to see one of them as their friends who will mother and comfort them while another one takes care of them.

This is also the way it is with me. It took me forever to explain this, but the reason it works better for me to have the nurse do the comforting is because when someone else does it I feel like it's me against them but if one of their own nurses do it I feel like I have one of them on my side and they are my friend and they will comfort me and help me through the pain the other nurse has to put me through when they stick me with needles. This also goes for if they cut on me with any sharp instruments awake or do biopsies. This is the way I want it and this is what I need and the nurses are the "comfort providers" so they need to meet the needs I ask them to meet as my "comfort providers".

> Hospice Patients Alliance
> Standards of Care-Nursing

Hospices must provide adequate nursing care to meet the needs of the patient. That is the law. "All nurses, including hospice nurses, are trained to provide care according to the accepted standards of practice within the nursing field. Standards of nursing practice and the "Code of Nurses" can be found by contacting your State's nursing association.

> Hospice Patients Alliance

The nurse's license authorizes her to perform professional assessments of her patients, create nursing plans of care, perform many skilled nursing procedures, provide all necessary aspects of nursing bedside care, and many other tasks. The nurse's license requires her to make sure the patient's needs are met."

> Hospice Patients Alliance

Did you see that? Hospice requires nurses to meet the "needs of their patients". It says the nurse's license requires her to make sure the "patient's needs are met".

I actually found a Comfort Behaviors Checklist on the Internet for Nurses observing their patients.
Number 11 on this list is how well a patient responds to "rubbing of an area", Number 14 on this list is how well the patient "accepts kindness", Number 15 on this list is how well the patient "likes touch/hand holding".
> This was on Dr. Katharine Kolcaba's website "Comfort Care in Nursing.

"Comfort is a concept that has a strong association with nursing. Nurses traditionally provide comfort to patients and their families through interventions that can be called comfort measures. The intentional comforting actions of nurses strengthen patients and their families. When patients and families are strengthened by actions of health care personnel (nurses), they can better engage in health seeking behaviors."
> Dr. Katharine Kolcaba, Comfort Care in Nursing

Remember how I said I always ask my nurses to "rub my head to calm me down and hold my hand through a needle stick". Notice what this says about Comfort Care in Nursing. The above is a comfort behaviors checklist by Dr. Katharine Kolcaba.
Notice I pointed out above that #11 on her list includes the patient's response to the "rubbing of an area" and that # 15 on her list includes the patient's response to how they like touch/hand holding.
See the connection. What I'm asking for is not wrong at all, it's a need I need met that you are already supposed to meet according to Dr. Katharine Kolcaba.

Here's more about the definition of what a nurse is and what they are supposed to do.

"For Centuries nurses have helped care for the sick and injured. The word "nurse" is from the Latin word nutrire, "to nourish" or "cherish".
>   The New Book of Knowledge, N13, page 409, 1970

"What a nurse does depends upon the needs of patients in the hospital units in which she works."
>   The New Book of Knowledge, N13, page 410, 1970

"Nursing is a career of service and dedication. It is a career that demands intelligence, dependability, "warmth", patience, and "an awareness of the feelings of others". In return, nursing offers the deep satisfaction of helping people in need and sharing closely in the joys and sorrows of others."
>   The New Book of Knowledge, N13, page 412, 1970

This quote even says nurses are supposed to "share closely in the joys and sorrows of others". It also says they are supposed to show "warmth" and "have awareness for the feelings of others", in other words their patients feelings, what they want and what they need.

"Nurses must really care about people and want to help them. People who are ill may feel alone and afraid, and nurses can give them confidence."
>   The New Book of Knowledge, N13, page 412, 1970

You can cheer them up and give them confidence, yes, but to really help them feel cared for and ease their pain and their fear and their need for love you also need to comfort them by giving them affection. That would be the hugs, the shoulder pats, the head rubs, the hand holds, etc.

You need to be willing to pat them on the shoulder and give them a hug and escort them to their room and say, "Hey, it's going to be okay. We're your friends. Come with me. We're going to take care of you." And give them a hug and a shoulder pat again when you have them sit on the patient bed and give them reassurance again. You could probably say something like, "I'm Lacy and I'm going to be your nurse today and we're going to help you. What do we need to do for you today? Can you tell me what you're in here for?"

Then, if it's something like a needle stick, or procedure, or anything else that might be scary for the patient, like I said, just keep showing them affection and saying, "It's okay. Don't be afraid. I'm going to be right here if you need me. You just tell me what you need me to do if you get scared and I'll do whatever you need me to do." I had a pre-op nurse at a hospital I used to go to that I went to procedures for probably 10 or 15 times in 10 years and she did this for me every time. My most recent lab tech and my newest family doctor's office also did this for me.

I've had several nurses be this way with me and everything was just fine. It's just these picky types that think they've got to be all proper acting as they say that won't do this for me. If they would just get off their soap box and cave in and do what I need them to do like these people did everything would go a lot better for everybody, me and them included. Believe it or not, it wasn't until the past couple of years I even ran into people like this. My old hospital had a turnover in nurses in two of their departments and they did not understand, but the ones that knew me before them did understand. If they would have stuck around, I would have never had to look anywhere else. Before the past couple of years, it was just hit and miss, once in a blue moon I'd have to go somewhere else and they wouldn't understand. Now, the very hospital that met all my needs for 10 years straight without complaining has gone the same way.

A different hospital I went to for a heart cath test two years ago promised Bertha they would meet every need I had on my lists I gave them. They started out meeting them the first two IV stick attempts but after I failed them twice because my veins collapsed, they suddenly got mean and rough with the needles and when I asked for more hugs and comfort they started complaining, "My nurses' have their rights! I'm not going to make them do anything they don't want to do! Not everybody is going to meet your needs!" They even told me that the one comforting me did not like my hugs (putting my right ear on their cheek).

They were ugly since and jabbed me hard with an IV in the left upper arm like they were giving me a shot instead of an IV at a straight shot instead of an angle, and the nurse that did this left my tourniquet on me an hour and a half before I noticed and I had to tell them myself they did this. They were even mean in the procedure room, one person right after another refusing to hug me. Only the 3rd and 4th one out of the five gave me a hug and I was in a panic state. If the 3rd one had not come in so jubilantly and said, "Sure!" when I asked her for a hug and acted pleased as pie to do it then they probably would have lost me or failed to get anything done right. Besides, when they did the actual procedure I was already asleep, had I not been and they would have refused to comfort me, the pain would have been so excruciating to me there's no way I would have got through it and disaster would have happened and they would have either seriously hurt me from my jerking in panic or lost me for sure. That was not a good move on their part and they could have caused me a heart attack and probably almost did. They also gave Bertha havoc over having to meet my needs when their top nurse already promised her that all my needs would be met two weeks earlier. I think when I told the hospital I normally go to what happened that even though some understood and felt bad about the way I was treated, I feel like all the new nurses hanging around started thinking, "Well, if they can get by with it, so can we. We don't want to meet his needs. If they don't have to meet his needs then neither do we. We have our rights too." But, if they had known what all their own school books in nursing had to say about the subject, they are required to comfort their patients and they are required to meet their patient's needs they would have seen things differently.

Just as it said in my books, it also said it in theirs, "It's not about the nurse's rights. It's the patient's rights that matter, and the patients needs come first above the nurses needs." Nursing is a "hands on" profession not a "hands off" profession. I think this is when things started going down hill and after the idea spread too far across the hospital, regardless of the few nurses that saw it my way, the rest of the nurses played follow the leader and gradually began to treat me the way the other hospital did and never met my needs again.

The right attitude of the nurse is not, "I'm the nurse, you're the patient, and so you just stand back" but "Hi. I'm you're nurse. I'm going to help you. You just hold on to me if you need to. Just let me know if there's anything I can do for you and I'll do what I can. I'll be right here for you." That's why we came over here to this new hospital, in hopes the nurses of this hospital would understand and meet my needs happily, like my ex-hospital did for me at one time for 10 years straight before they turned on me. I just want doctor's offices and a hospital that will be the same way with me my original nurses were with me before they all quit their jobs and the way the Pre-Op people still were with me when I left their facility. They met every need on my list.

My favorite pre-op nurse always gave me hugs and always rubbed my head to calm me down and held my hand to do an IV stick. Sometimes I did really well. Other times I still screamed in excruciating pain. One time they thought they had the needle in and everything seemed to be going unusually well, but then the IV tech said, "I'm sorry. I can't get the needle to thread. We're going to have to do it again. We're going to have to stick you again. I'm sorry." I said, "Please. Don't make me do it again." My favorite pre-op nurse said, "I'm sorry honey. We have to do this." She rubbed my head again and this time I screamed in excruciating pain at the top of my lungs." I told her, "I'm sorry. I didn't mean to mess up or be difficult for you." My favorite Pre-Op nurse then said, "Don't worry about me. I'm here for you."

When I was in the hospital in October 2012 for chest pain and the inpatient nurses back then had to readjust my IV it took five chipper acting, cheerful female nurses to rethread the needle that was loose in my vein and of course I went ballistic on them. I was so sorry I gave them so much trouble and I said, "I'm sorry I'm so hard to deal with and that you had so much trouble reinserting my IV." Then, one of them said, "I want to tell you something. You may have trouble getting through IVs and other invasive stuff, but that is a far cry from what we have to put up with from patients who have no pain yet gripe and complain over every little trivial thing. I want you to know you are the most well behaved patient we have ever had and I really appreciate it."

Unfortunately, the girls that did this for me that understood me all quit their jobs and got other jobs at other clinics and nursing homes and rehab centers and the like. The girls that replaced them in the past year or two were not very understanding of me and were not very fond of having to show affection to their patients.

They were just there for the check and I was shocked because the girls before them were so much more caring and compassionate and comforting and understanding and never had any trouble giving me hugs or comforting me like these new people did. These new people were stoic acting.

One of my Radiology techs went to help comfort me through B12 shots and blood tests at the hospital the same way my favorite PreOp nurse helped comfort me through my IVs. One day this girl got tired of having to do this for me. After I asked several of the other girls I liked to do this for me if she didn't want to she went and told all the rest of them not to cave in and meet my needs because she wanted to straighten me out so I'd quit acting like a 5-year-old. So, then, not only had ER and Inpatient had a turnover in nurses who did not understand me, but now they had turned on me too, and a little bit later they said nobody there was ever going to hug me or comfort me ever again. One lady asked Bertha to try to get a Children's Hospital to take me because the nurses there were not equipped to meet my needs because they were not trained to take care of Autistic Adults. Then, she thought they would think the Children's Hospitals would think I was too old and needed to go to a hospital that took care of special needs adults.

I tried a doctor's office and hospital someone claimed worked with Autistic adults but they turned on me too. That's why I decided to find someone somewhere else that would work with me the way I am and meet my needs that I have without complaint.

I've found several new doctors who are willing to meet my needs including their nurses so I hope it all works out.

You know how I wish that I could feel like my nurses care about me and want to help me and how the ones that understand me have given me confidence to go on. Look what this quote says up here. That's exactly what they're supposed to do.

"Nursing is also good preparation for raising a family. Nurses learn about health, illness, child care, and relationships among people."
>   The New Book of Knowledge, N13, page 412, 1970

Remember what I said about treating your patients like your own children, that's why this quote above says that nursing is a good preparation for raising a family. You get a lot of practice by giving comfort to your patients.

Here are a few quotes about how hospitals are supposed to be with their patients. That would mean the nurses that work in these hospitals.

"A Hospital is an institution for the treatment and care of persons who need medical attention. Night and day, the members of the hospital staff work as a well-drilled team to provide for the comfort and health of patients."
>   The World Book Encyclopedia, H, page 332, 1967

"In the hospital corridors, white-uniformed nurses move quickly and quietly from room to room, bringing comfort to their patients."
>   The World Book Encyclopedia, H, page 332, 1967

"A modern hospital is designed to provide for a patient's comfort as well as his health."
>   The World Book Encyclopedia, H, page 332, 1967

Did you just see that? It says a modern hospital is designed to provide for the patient's comfort as well as his health.

"Professional Services staff consists of hospital personnel directly concerned with the care of patients."

> The World Book Encyclopedia, H, page 332, 1967

"The word hospital comes from the Latin word hospitium, which means a house or institution for guests."

> The World Book Encyclopedia, H, page 335, 1967

Did you notice something here?

 It didn't say the hospital is a place for a bunch of professionals to do business with each other and break business deals.
 It says it is a house or institution for guests which means it's more personal than that.

"The hospital offers a large variety of careers for persons interested in helping the sick. Those who like to help other people will find hospital work a good life. This work is hard and demanding on a person's time and energy. However, there is compensation for all the day to day problems and hardships – the conviction that this work is essential to humanity."

> The World Book Encyclopedia, H, page 335, 1967

"The emphasis on comfort and the role it plays in health care has changed in the last 10 decades. From 1900 to 1929, comfort was the central focus and moral imperative of nursing: from 1930 to 1959, comfort was considered a strategy for achieving fundamental requirements of nursing care: and from 1960 to 1980, comfort fell out of favor, to become only a minor aspect of nursing, and was significant only to people who received no medical treatment. During the last 3 decades, comfort has been relegated to end-of-life care where it is equated with the simplest aspects of care, which could be just as easily provided by nonprofessional caregivers."

> Chia-Chia, Lin, PhD, RN
> School of Nursing, Taiwan
> Comfort: A Value Forgotten in Nursing-Lin, Chia-Chia PhD, RN
> Cancer, Nursing: November/December 2010-Volume 33-Issue 6-pp409-410

"Today, as always, comfort remains a substantive need throughout our oncology nurses play an important role in promoting comfort through their lives."

> Chia-Chia, Lin, PhD, RN
> School of Nursing, Taiwan
> Comfort: A Value Forgotten in Nursing-Lin, Chia-Chia PhD, RN
> Cancer, Nursing: November/December 2010-Volume 33-Issue 6-pp409-410

"Comfort is not a novel idea and has been cited by prestigious and cancer patients. In conclusion, comfort should not be relegated to end-of-life care. There is a powerful need for an increase in translational research to promote comfort in every stage of patient care. When comfort is emphasized in nursing care and when promoting comfort becomes an important core value of nursing, I believe that nurses will gain more respect from their patients, the families of patients, and our colleagues in the field of medicine."

> Chia-Chia, Lin, PhD, RN
> School of Nursing, Taiwan
> Comfort: A Value Forgotten in Nursing-Lin, Chia-Chia PhD, RN
> Cancer, Nursing: November/December 2010-Volume 33-Issue 6-pp409-410

There it is again. This doesn't say nurses aren't required to comfort their patients and it's not in their job description to do so. It says that nurses are required to comfort their patients but they have gotten out of line over a period of time and relegated comforting their patients to only being covered by end of life care. If you notice, they say, this should not be so but that all stages of patient care and not just end of life care should comfort their patients. They also point out that when comfort is emphasized in nursing care and promoting comfort becomes an important core value of nursing like it once was that nurses will gain more respect from their patients, the families of their patients, and their colleagues in the field of medicine. I can tell you I did, while they were willing to comfort me.

To Nurse Means To Nurture   Brian Evans

When I was a kid and nurses were mean to me they had to chase
me all over the hospital to get anything done and I had a bad
opinion of nurses until the day came when I ran into nice nurses
that would be nice and comfort me and be as gentle as they
possibly could with their needles.

Now, that some nurses wish to refuse to comfort me, I feel like
running again and don't feel comfortable sticking around unless
they do comfort me through my procedures and when I go see the
doctor as well.

On the movie, "Facing Death" I noted all of the following
situations where a nurse comforted their patients and how they did
it. I counted nine instances in which they occurred and here's what
they did.

In the first instance, a female nurse rubbed a male patients' head at
the beginning of the movie. You could also say they stroked his
head because they moved their hand across his head petting him on
the head in the same way you would do for your dog or your cat or
your baby.

In the second instance, another female nurse rubbed a woman
patient's head in this same manner and then pushed the skin up
above her eye with her thumb and rubbed her forehead with her
thumb and then rubbed her head again with her hand.
In other words, she stroked the top of the lady's head with her hand
continually like you would do for your dog or your cat or your
baby.

In the third instance, the female nurse that comforted the lady
patient in the second instances went back and rubbed the lady
patient's head again and stroked the top of her head with her hand
continually.

In the fourth instance, another female nurse held a patient's hand
while another nurse pulled him on his side.

They put a blue pad thing under his back and then stroked his head, rubbed his head to calm him down and actually straightened his hair to the side with her hand as she comforted him.

In the fifth instance, another female nurse rubbed the top of another patient's head.
In the sixth instance, another female nurse patted a guy patient on the head when he said he was scared of having a catheter put in and said they didn't have to do it if he didn't want them to.

In the seventh instance, a female nurse put her hand on a male patient's head and then rubbed his head.

In the eighth instance, a female nurse put her hand on a male patient's shoulder, rubbed it a minute, and then held his hand and rubbed his head.

In the ninth instance, another female nurse held the same male patient's hand and moved her hand across his upper arm to comfort him.

And some nurses tell me they think that's not in their job description.

Why can't they do this for everybody? Do they have to be dying in order for a nurse to comfort them?

These people that they did this for were not even mentally disabled as I am. These people were normal acting people in a normal everyday hospital being taken care of by everyday hospital nurses, and yet some nurses think that it is out of line to do this for me, when not only do I need this kind of comforting care but I need it all the more than the normal patient because I have a mental disability causing me to have childlike needs which causes me to need these things all the more than any other patient would.
You saw the comment made by the nurse with the PhD above. She said that comfort should not be relegated to end of life care but should be promoted in every stage of patient care.

She also said that nurses would gain more respect from their patients and their patients' families when comfort was promoted and became an important core in nursing care as it should be. That's the way it should be. That's what I need. I need your comfort when I am under your care.

"Most nurses work in hospitals, where they help comfort and care for people who are sick, injured, or recovering from surgery."
World Book Encyclopedia, Number 14, N, page 618, 2006

See, this quote comes out and says it. Nurses comfort the people that come to them, not shun them away and say, "I'm just here to do business. I can't get too personal. I'm a professional. That's not appropriate." That's bogus.
That's like a deacon in a church that says he's going to run things because "he's the deacon" when in fact, a deacon is a "servant" or "slave" that goes and visits "the fatherless and the widows". Not all deacons are like this, but if the ones that thought this knew what a deacon was, they'd get off their soap box in a minute and wind up eating humble pie. That's the same way with nurses. You're not an executive of a firm. You're a caretaker of a patient and you are there to serve your patients with comfort and full compassion. If you realized that, you might feel different too and then think on the right wavelength to do your job compassionately.

"Nursing offers daily satisfaction to those who have a genuine desire to help others."
World Book, Number 14, N, page 619, 2006

I understand for some odd reason, some nurses are scared of lists when it comes to a patient giving them a list of the accommodations they need them to meet. Many of them act as if they think it's horrible that a patient would even ask for the things they do.

They don't understand why they don't just take it like a man like everyone else and quit being such a big baby, either that or they have some wild outlandish idea that there is some horrible reasoning behind their list when all they are doing is asking them to meet the very needs they are supposed to meet if it is what the patient wants and needs them to do.

Did you know that some patients are told to give their nurses one of their lists of needs so they'll know how to deal with them?

So, why do nurses get so upset about a patient giving them a list of their needs and asking for them to meet their needs when there have been some patients that have been told to give them a list of needs?

I would like to show you something I found in a book called "The Fearless Caregiver" that says this very thing on pages 50 and 51 when getting Home Health Aides to come out and take care of your loved ones.

You know what it says? Be completely honest about your needs.

You're probably thinking, "Whoa! Where did that come from? I didn't know I was supposed to take inventory of their needs and ask them to tell me what they are and meet them?"

Well, you are. I don't know how nurses always seem to miss this these days. They always knew better than to question these things until the recent past.
Check this out. Here's what things this book says to do when preparing a Home Health Aid to deal with a loved one, and I guarantee you that goes for a nurse as well. Here goes.

1. Be completely honest about your needs.
2. Overcome any embarrassment or guilt associated with describing why you need help and what kind of help you need.

Note, it also says on #2: "Remember that you are dealing with professionals that have helped a variety of clients. They are experienced in meeting the needs of people just like you."

3. State your preferences from the start.

Note: #3 also says, "The best way to get what you want is to be specific. Give a detailed request to the agency so that the aid it sends will meet your needs."

Did you catch that? It says to "be specific about what you want and send a detailed request to the agency". Why? It says to do this so that the aid will "meet your needs."

4. Give feedback to the agency on a timely basis.

Note in the book #4 also says that if you are not happy with the aide the agency can send you a different aide.

"The Fearless Caregiver", Gary Barg, Today's Caregiver Magazine,
       Capital Books Incorporated, Caregiver Media Group, 2001

Now you guys see why I write you so much.

Now let's take my situation and narrow this down. I don't like male nurses because I was tortured by males when I was a kid with needles. The serious trended female nurses did the same thing in my childhood and adulthood.
The chipper acting female nurses, whenever I actually managed to get them for my nurses were very sweet and compassionate and willing to comfort me the way I asked them to comfort me through needle sticks and gave me hugs also as I asked and all went well.

If we take this above situation and we take my request for chipper acting female nurses only, we can see that just as in the case of the person getting the home health aide in the book I am letting the nurses know ahead of time which nurses I am comfortable with taking care of me.

And, like the individual receiving home health who is requesting
home health aides and nurses that best suit their personal needs I
am also requesting nurses in the doctor's offices and hospitals who
best suit my personal needs. And just as it is okay for them to list
the needs they have and request the home health aids that best suit
these needs they have, it is also okay for me to request nurses that
best suit the needs I have stated on my own list of needs. There's
nothing wrong with what I am asking, and technically, the nurses
are already supposed to meet these needs for me anyway.
And from what I have seen in movies, including true story movies,
and also from my own personal experiences, there are nurses that
do the very things for other people on a regular basis that I am
asking them to do for me, so what I am asking of them is nothing
amiss.

As far as the writing things I also found these quotes about
patient's writing their nurses.

"Therapeutic Writing – a treatment technique in which patients are
asked to write an account of the traumatic event and their
emotional responses to it."
> The Gale Encyclopedia of Medicine, 5th Edition, page 572,
> Yolameg Books, 2010

"There are four main branches of nursing, adult, child, mental
health, and 'learning disability'".
> Blacks Medical Dictionary, 42nd Edition, Dr. Harvey
> Marcovitch, 2010

Since I am autistic and have a learning disability, in addition to
having the childlike emotional needs I have, sometimes it's easier
to write down for you what I need than to have to explain all of it
to you. I can tell you verbally what most of my needs are but I get
easily stumped when I talked to people and sometimes get my
message jumbled when I try to tell you what I need or have a hard
time knowing how to say or ask something important.

Sometimes it's hard to remember things the doctor wants to know if I haven't' seen them in a month or so, so it's easier to write it down for them. And, I always like to write lists to tell nurses what my needs are so they can meet them and know what to do for me. Now you guys see why I write you so much.

Nurses may feel like they have to go way out of their way to help me and wonder why I have to be so much trouble but notice what this next statement says I found in the World Book Encyclopedia from 2006.

"A nurse must like people and want to help them and must also have self-reliance and good judgment. Patience, tact, honesty, responsibility, and ability to work easily with others are valuable traits. Good health is another must."
     World Book, Number 14, N, page 619, 2006

You see, they're supposed to like working with people like me and want to help them and have patience with them regardless of how trying they may be to you.

"In all schools of nursing, classroom work or theory is interwoven with practice. Clinical experience, or practice, means the time that the student spends in learning to spend with different types of patients."
     World Book, Number 14, N, page 619, 2006

I would definitely pass for a different type of patient that most patients. I have oversensitivity to pain and a fear of needles, and I have a dire need for comfort by means of affection, hugging, hand holding, head rubs, shoulder rubs, etc.

The needle sticks are so painful to me that a shot and a blood test feel like a steak knife to me, an IV feels like a butcher knife to me, and a catheter feels like a sword being run through me. I have to put Lidocaine/Prilocaine 2.5% cream on the site of the stick one hour before being stuck just to knock out the pain.

Sometimes it knocks it all out. Other times it only knocks some of the pain out, which can still mean it will be excruciating if it doesn't work as well that time.

I am a very needy person because I need the motherly comfort of a chipper acting female nurse to give me hugs and rub my head to calm me down and hold my hand through needle sticks and I am afraid of male nurses, doctors, and techs as well as serious trended female nurses because all these tortured me with needles when I was a kid. The serious trended female nurses even tortured me in adulthood. The chipper acting, cheery, motherly female nurses are the only ones I am comfortable with and they are usually willing to comfort me the way I want to be comforted. It wasn't until recently that any of them felt different because they thought they were somehow above comforting their patients, but the ones who did not feel this way about it always comforted me the way I wanted comforted. I don't know what's wrong with everybody else. A bunch of nurses got on a "what they think is proper" kick and "forgot they were caretakers" that were supposed to take care of their patients by comforting them as well as doing their technical nursing job. I think they overlooked some of the things they were supposed to learn about bedside manner when they took their classes. They probably just skimmed over it and read the rest and just thought who cares about that, I want to know how to perform my job by learning the technically correct way to give a shot or blood test or sew someone together. What good is that without comfort? Nursing without love for the patient and caring about their needs is not nursing at all. Nursing is nurturing your patients as you do your job so they can feel comforted anytime they come to see you. You're there to make them feel better not worse. Please try to see where I'm coming from and try to understand the importance of comforting your patients.

These quotes I have found from encyclopedias, internet references, and even college medical school books are telling you the same thing I am saying, so please here my plea, and comfort me and all your other patients that come to you.

Here are some more quotes clarifying all the more that my plea for comfort is not in vain. Please keep reading and try to understand. I really need this and so do others.

"In selecting a nursing home, it is important to match both the medical and psychological needs of a person with the recourses of the care giving institution. Nursing homes also should provide for the psychological needs of their residents."
        World Book, Number 14, N, page 620, 2006

"Nursing students study such subjects as anatomy, chemistry, nutrition, pharmacology, physiology, psychology, and sociology, as well as the fundamentals of nursing care. They learn to care for the sick by working in the nursing laboratory. Frequently, the students practice on one another."
        World Book, Number 14, N, page 619, 2006

You would think with these nurses practicing on each other and seeing how much pain it puts them in to give each other IVs and whatever else they do to each other that is painful that they would understand what pain their patients are feeling when they do this to them.

I just found the following quote in one of my medical assisting books that proves some patients can't handle pain well.

"A patient who has excruciating pain will require a larger dose of analgesic than a patient who has intermittent pain."
        Clinical Skills and Assisting Techniques for the Medical
        Assistant, Sharon M. Zakus, RN, BA, MS, CMA, page 248,
        1988.

This proves that there are some patients out there with oversensitivity to pain and I am one of them.
If there were not any patients like this around this comment would not be in this nurse's book written for Medical Assistants.

The following comment was made for medical assistants assisting doctors with minor surgeries in a doctor's office.

"Remember, any surgical procedure is an invasion into body parts not normally interfered with; and although it may be a minor surgical procedure, it often does not appear minor to the patient. Many patients are somewhat anxious, nervous, or concerned about what is going to happen. The medical assistant can and must help the patient relax and ally any fears of apprehensions. On arrival of the patient in the office, greet and usher the patient into the treatment room. Attend to the patient's needs for "comfort" and communication, and give emotional support and reassurance. The best of care can be enhanced by evaluating every patient and situation individually."

> Clinical Skills and Assisting Techniques for the Medical Assistant, Sharon M. Zakus, RN, BA, MS, CMA, page 161, 1988.

This quote talking to the medical assistant says that they "can and must" help the patient relax and ally any apprehensions. The way you do that for me is to talk to me gently in a cheerful voice, give me a hug and then be ready to rub my head to calm me down and hold my hand through a needle stick when another chipper acting female nurse does the stick. This quote is saying you should be more concerned about how much you might be hurting your patients with some of your devices that seem like no big deal for you to use but is a big deal for them because they may be in excruciating pain and need your comfort for sure.

"Nursing is a profession the members of which provide auxiliary care to the sick and disabled under the direction of physician's or other medical specialists."

> Funk and Wagnall's Encyclopedia, page 6243, The Universal Standard Encyclopedia, 1988.

Some doctors and nurses don't want to deal with me because of my disability because it would mean they would have to baby me to death but this is what I need. This quote is saying here they are to provide auxiliary care to the sick "and the disabled" so you need to be willing to take care of me being disabled and care for me comforting me the way I need to be comforted and not the way you decide you want to comfort me.

"Most nursing schools require the candidates be graduated from high school and have two years of science as well as good health and a personality suited to the demands of service to the sick."
  Funk and Wagnall's Encyclopedia, page 6243, The
  Universal Standard Encyclopedia, 1958.

"Among the rewards of nursing are the challenges it offers. A badly injured person may need immediate and expert care. Medicines and equipment must be rushed to the patient's bedside. The family must be comforted and the doctor must be given a detailed report on the patient's condition. A nurse's greatest reward often is the knowledge that his or her skill has helped to relieve suffering or to save a life."
  World Book, Number 14, N, page 619, 2006.

This even says the family must be comforted.

"The well-being of patients is of first importance to nurses. They take time to reassure worried patients and boost the patient's morale. Nurses are taught to recognize and understand patients' needs and provide emotional support as well as physical care."
  World Book, Number 14, N, page 617, 2006

You can see by reading this you need to encourage your patients and try to cheer them up and be willing to physically comfort them to make them feel better.

Here's the same quote expanded in a newer version of the same encyclopedia 8 years later:

"The well being of patients is of first importance to nurses. RNs are taught to recognize and understand patients' needs. They provide emotional support as well as physical care, taking time to reassure worried patients and boost their moral. Each type of patient has special needs, requiring nurses with specialized knowledge or training. As a result, hospital nurses typically choose an area of specialty just as most doctors develop a specialty.

Nurses' specialties range from basic primary care to fields requiring highly developed technical skills. Patients often get most of their direct care through nurses."

World Book, N-O, Volume 414, 616, 2014

"Nurse's aides give important social and emotional support to patients as the registered nurses may not have enough time to spend with the patients. Nurse's aides help by answering patient calls; feeding, washing, and walking patients; and recording vital signs and other indications of a patient's care. If a patient's aides go along they may help support patients during treatment of help move them onto or off of beds and stretchers."

World Book, N-O, Volume 14, page 616, 2014

"Most nurses work in hospitals where they comfort and care for people who are sick, injured, or are recovering from surgery."

World Book, N-O, Volume 14, 616, 2014

See. There it is again. And, this is a 2014 encyclopedia we're talking about. It even says nurses are supposed to comfort their patients.

"Nursing offers satisfaction to those who desire to help. A nurse must like people and want to help them."

World Book, N-O, Volume 14, 616, 2014

See, this says you're supposed to want to help your patients, not just see them in to do your thing and then send them out. Help them. Nursing is supposed to be for those who desire to help their patients not for people who just want to do their job and get a check. It's for people who like helping the people they work with. "Good nursing consists in securing as much physical comfort as possible for the patient in rendering prompt first aid in emergencies that may arise, and in soothing and cheering the patient's mind."

Victor Robinson, Ph.C., M.D., Modern Home Physician, Wise, 1968

Even a doctor said nurses need to comfort their patients in this quote, and he said physical comfort, but it's from 1968. Still, all the same, they still need to comfort their patients no matter when this quote was made.

"Nursing is also good preparation for raising a family. Nurses learn about health, illness, child care, and relationships among people."
>   The New Book of Knowledge, N13, page 412, 1970

Like I said, you treat your patients like children and it better equips you to take care of children and show them the compassion they need as well as your patients. It teaches you a lesson in how to love people, a very important lesson to learn in raising a family. You need to care for your patients not just see them as a number. You are their "caretaker" or "caregiver". Give them the care they need, don't just do your thing and send them away. Comfort them. Treat them like your own children.

To Nurse means to nurture. Nurture in the dictionary also means nourish.

I like a spelling thesaurus gadget a friend gave me. I don't really have trouble spelling. I just play with it for kicks to get meanings of words. According to this thesaurus gadget a friend at bingo gave me, the word nurse means "to act as a parent to." I've been looking for this definition the whole time. That's what I thought it meant.

So, you see, nurses are actually supposed to treat their patients as if they were their own children and provide the same love and affection toward their patients as they would their own child.

To those who wish to be nurses, you are not just taking on a profession where you stick patients with a bunch of needles and help with surgeries and then receive a paycheck for it. You are acting as a parent to these people. You are their caretaker and you are actually supposed to treat these people that are your patients like they are your children while they are under your care.

Anything you would do for your child from a comforting standpoint needs to be done for your patients. That's why I believe one of the people I copied the quote of in my book said that being a nurse is a great teaching tool for how to raise your kids. I think they meant that you were supposed to comfort them and console them in their fear and pain with great compassion. And, they did say in their quote that you are supposed to comfort your patients, by the way. That means if they need you to pat them on the shoulder, or give them a hug, or rub their head to calm them down and hold their hand you need to do so you have to do this for them. You would do this for your kids wouldn't you? Your patients need you to do the same for them no matter what their age. In case you think I am the only one emphasizing age one of the people I quoted said that comfort should not be left to end of life care but that people of all ages should be comforted by their nurses.

So, you see, nurses were supposed to comfort their patients all along. It's just that some of the nurses in the bigger hospitals have let pride get in the way of their jobs as comforters, and have stopped meeting their patients' needs, abandoning the earlier practices of nursing where comfort was the main key. Instead they think of themselves as someone above having to meet the needs of their patients, like they think they are business executives, when in fact, they are caregivers that are responsible for meeting the needs of their patients, including comforting and consoling them in their fear and pain.

So, please remember to reevaluate your responsibility as a nurse and remember that comforting your patients is the key to good patient care.

By the way, one of your own medical professionals also made this quote almost exactly. I'm just confirming it. You didn't know I knew all this did you? Please make sure to remember to comfort me and all your patients when they come your way.

As I said, any nurse that is unwilling to comfort their patients like a mother would comfort her child or baby should not be a nurse and should find a different profession to work in.

Please consider this insight when you try to decide whether to pursue a career in nursing as this is very important to the patient and their emotional needs need met including the need to be physically comforted and touched as well as their medical physical needs. They need your hugs and your shoulder pats and your head rubs and your hand holds. That's what nurses are for. They used to do it all the time. So, please, like the person in the one quote said begin to comfort your patients again and you will gain more respect from your patients and their families as well as your own colleagues again. Please, let comfort thrive again as it did before. The requirement to do so and the need for it never changed, just the idea the nurses have that they should have to do it is changed. You're still supposed to do this. Why do you think I found quotes all the way to 2014 saying so?

So, please, have mercy on me and everyone else and comfort your patients again the way you used to comfort them and not the way you do with this non shallot stuff that isn't even comfort. Comfort them the way they want you to comfort them and need you to comfort them and comfort them the way you would your own children and treat them like they're your children. This is what patients need and I need this worse than ever because I am autistic and crave touch and need a lot of affection from all those who work with me especially when I am scared. Wouldn't you rather comfort me the way I want you to comfort me and need you to comfort me instead of having to worry about chasing me all over the hospital like the nurses had to do when I was a kid?

When nurses starting meeting my requests and doing what I needed by comforting me in the way I asked them to and not how they decided they wanted to comfort me but in the way I wanted and needed to be comforted that's when things went well for all them and me. And when I tell nurses what I want them to do to comfort me if I give them a list of my needs, those aren't just wants, those are genuine needs.
When the few other nurses out there I ran into in the past couple of years starting complaining about their rights and not wanting to comfort me, that's when I started running the other way again.

So, if you want me to do anything for you, comfort me the way I am asking you to comfort me and give me hugs, rub my head to calm me down and hold my hand through needle sticks, and only give me the chipper acting cheery female nurses who have the motherly personality to do these things the way I need them done. Also, remember my pain. I need to put Lidocaine/Prilocaine 2.5% cream on the site of the stick one hour before you even do these needle sticks. Don't forget, I can't handle pain as well as most patients, so if you decide to come at me with a catheter or tube or wish to do an invasive procedure on me, please put me completely to sleep before you do so. Please, have mercy on me and do all this for me. This is what I need and I cannot handle it any other way. Please. You're supposed to do this for your patients and this is what I need. Be sure to comfort me and all your patients that come your way and treat them with love and compassion and comfort. Your patients need you and they need your love. Show it to them. Please.

Here are some examples from true story nursing books about how nurses comfort their patients to show you there are nurses out there that do comfort you the way I am asking you to comfort me:

In the book, "Nurses at Work" by Karen Latchana Kenney you will notice on page 25, it says that nurses need to be "caring" and "kind", and it shows a picture of a nurse looking sweetly at a girl in bed with her hand on the girl's head, on top of her hair even, not her forehead, even if she is taking her temperature.
I believe this lady is showing comfort to this girl out of the goodness of her own heart because she is a compassionate nurse. And, this is a kid's book, yes, but it is a non-fiction kid's book about nurses so that facts found in this book are very real.

On page 5 of this book you will also notice a nurse place her hand on a boy's upper back while she takes his blood pressure and temperature while she smiles joyfully at him.

I think she is comforting him too by gently touching his upper back for consolation while she takes his blood pressure.

> Nurses at Work by Karen Latchana Kenney, Content
> Consultant: Judy Stepan-Norris, PhD, Professor or
> Sociology, University of California, Irvine, Magic Wagon,
> 2010

In the book, "Community Helpers- Nurses" you will notice on page 9 of this "non-fiction" kid's book a lady nurse is bending over to gently touch a senior lady on the shoulder that has a gas mask on as she lays in her patient bed in the emergency room. They may have been putting this lady to sleep or giving her oxygen. This nurse smiles sweetly at her while she touches her shoulder and you can tell by the look in her eyes she cares for the lady and wants to meet her needs and comfort her.

On page 21 of this same book, it says, "Patients are the first concern of nurses. Nurses are taught to see a patient's illness. They are also taught to 'see their feelings'. They want patients to be happy and healthy."

> Community Helpers: Nurses by Dee Ready, Ready
> Consultant: Marie   Griffin, RN, C, Member of the
> American Nurses Association, Bridgestone Book, Capstone
> Press, 1997

In the book, "Florence Nightingale–Demi" Florence Nightingale comments, "Nursing is one of the Fine Arts; I had almost said the finest of the Fine Arts."

> Florence Nightingale, Una and the Lion, 1868
> Florence Nightingale: Demi, Henry Holt and Company,
> LLC. 2014

You will notice in the middle of this same book there is a page with a picture of a nurse holding the hand of a lady patient in bed and handing her a cup of water as well.

> Florence Nightingale: Demi, Henry Holt and Company,
> LLC, 2014

In the book, "Florence Nightingale: The Lady of the Lamp" it is stated that Florence Nightingale "paused many times bending down to place a cool hand on a forehead or to whisper soothing words."

> Florence Nightingale, The Lady of the Lamp by Kay Barnham, Raintree Steck-Vaughn Publishers, 2003

Now we are getting personal, but we're supposed to. We're nurses. We're the comfort providers, remember.

Florence Nightingale considers herself to be a "mother" to her patients. She feels bad about leaving the men she took care of when she went home and left them in the Crimean grave. She makes the following comment concerning this, "Oh my poor men who endured so patiently. I feel I have been such a bad mother to you to come home and leave you lying in the Crimean grave. Seventy three percent from disease alone – who thinks of that now?"

> Florence Nightingale, The Lady and the Lamp, page 29
> Florence Nightingale, 1856 Kay Barnham, Raintree Steck-Vaughn Publishers, 2003

And some of you nurses think you're too big for that because your professional and this is too personal for you. Try to learn from the best. We're talking about the most popular nurse in History here that felt this way. She was very emotional and considered herself to be a mother to her patients.

Florence Nightingale made this comment about nurses.

"No man, not even a doctor, ever gives any other definition of what a nurse should be than this – 'devoted and obedient'. This definition would do just as well for a porter. It might even do for a horse."

> Florence Nightingale, The Lady and the Lamp, page 33
> Stock Vaughn Company, 2003

Speaking of a compassionate nurse, look what I found in this book, "Gentle Annie: The True Story of a Civil War Nurse".

Annie had men falling dead left and right off of horses she tried to catch while they were wounded and still alive. This is what the book says she did to the one she spoke to for a moment that then fell dead: "Blinking the tears from her eyes, she closed his gently. Then she touched his cheek with the palm of her hand the way his own mother might have done if she had found him here."

> Gentle Annie: The True Story of a Civil War Nurse,
> page 86, Mary Francis Shura, Scholastic Inc., 1991

Now that's comfort and compassion.

This nurse wrote letters for some of these military men to their wives that had difficulty writing for themselves and she even wiped the soup off a man's mustache he wrote letters for.

> Gentle Annie: The True Story of a Civil War Nurse,
> Page 100, Mary Francis Shura, Scholastic, Inc., 1991

Throughout this book Annie is continually moved with compassion toward the men she took care of when she saw them wounded and tried to comfort them. On the back cover of this book there is even a comment at the end that says, "She was beloved by the men of her regiment, writing letters for them to their loved ones, and comforting them in their pain." The lady's real name stated at the end of the book is Anna B. Ethridge.

> Gentle Annie, The True Story of a Civil War Nurse,
> Mary Francis, Shura, Scholastic, Inc., 1991

Sounds like a nice nurse, huh. So, now, why can't you be that way as well?

In the book, "Clara Barton and Her Victory over Fear", Clara Barton took care of her brother when she was eleven years old. He wanted only his devoted Clara at his bedside. "He had been my ideal from earliest memory", Clara said. "I was distressed beyond measure at his condition. I had been his little protégé', his companion, and in his nervous wretchedness he clung to me."

> "Clara Barton and Her Victory Over Fear" by Robert
> Quakenbush, page 15, Simon & Schuster Books for Young
> Adults, 1995.

"Clara Barton actually quit school for two years just to take care of him. He finally tried a clinic that promoted steam baths and other types of water cures and his health was restored in three weeks. If you will notice, she puts her hand to his head holding a wet rag to her brother's head while she holds his arm with her other hand."
"Clara Barton and Her Victory over Fear", page 15

Now, you're probably going to say that's because it is her brother. In that case, get this, Clara went onto the battlefield to nurse people and nothing stopped her on her mission.
She had to dodge gunshots just to help the soldiers. Once she stopped to give a fallen soldier a drink of water and she "cradled him in her arms" but unfortunately a bullet passed under her arm hitting him and killed him.
"Clara Barton and Her Victory over Fear",
Robert Quakenbush, page 24 Simon & Schuster Books for Young Readers, 1995

"Many things frightened Clara as a child. When she was barely two and a half years old she was terrified by a snake she saw slithering near the stoop where she was playing. Another time, she wandered into the barn where some farm hands were about to butcher an ox. One of them butchered an ox and she fainted. She recalled an experience during her childhood where a relative died and a thunder shower approached right when they were about to have a funeral and she wound up not attending because of it. Looking up from a window, Clara saw massive rifts of clouds rolling in the sky and lightening darting among them like blazing fires. 'My Terrors transformed those rising, rolling clouds into a whole heaven full of angry rams, marching down on me', said Clara and she began screaming. David, her brother, rushed to her side to reassure her but the memory of how frightened she had been would be with her forever. Because of all this, from an early age, Clara showed empathy for the suffering of others which became part of her character."
"Clara Barton and Her Victory over Fear",
Robert Quakenbush, page 24, Simon & Shuster Books for Young Readers, 1995

"Clara was shy and appeared without gloves one Sunday just as the family was leaving for church. She told her mother the gloves were wore out and burst into tears when her mother asked her why she didn't ask for new ones."
>"Clara Barton and Her Victory over Fear",
> Robert Quakenbush, page 24, Simon & Schuster Books for Young Readers, 1995

"Clara discovered the Red Cross while in Geneva to recuperate and when she returned to the United States she was eager to form a branch of the Red Cross in America that would aid victims of disaster in peacetime as well as in war."
>"Clara Barton and Her Victory over Fear",
>Robert Quakenbush, page 16 Simon and Schuster Books for Young Readers, 1995

"Clara Barton founded the American Red Cross Society on May 21, 1881 and was elected president of the society."
>"Clara Barton and Her Victory over Fear",
>Robert Quakenbush, page 16, Simon and Schuster Books for Young Readers, 1995

"Caring for her brother helped Clara learn how to take care of sick people."
>American Lives: Clara Barton", page 10, Elizabeth Raum, Heinemann Library, 2004

"President Abraham Lincoln told people that Barton would help them search for missing soldiers."
>American Lives: Clara Barton, page 20, Elizabeth Raum, Heinemann Library, 2004

Notice on the cover of the book, "Clara Barton and Her Victory over Fear" they show Clara Barton holding a cup of water up to a soldier's mouth for him to drink and she puts her other arm around his shoulder."

What a compassionate woman this is to show love for her fellow soldiers and give comfort to those in distress that needed her help who were soldiers.

This is a wonderful act indeed and should be an act of compassion among all nurses toward their patients as this woman was.

"Clara was known as the "Daughter of the Regiment" in the 21st Massachusetts Regiment."
>DK Biography: Clara Barton, A Photographic Story of a
>Life, page 58, Steven Krensky, DK Publishing, 2011

"At the end of 1864, Clara was made the superintendent of the Department of Nurses for the army massed along the James River in West Virginia."
>DK Biography: Clara Barton, A Photographic Story of a
>Life, page 63, Steven Krensky, DK Publishing, 2011

"She was perhaps the most perfect incarnation of mercy the modern world has known."
>The Detroit Free Press, DK Biography: Clara Barton, A
>Photographic Story of a Life, page 115, Steven Krensky,
>DK Publishing, 2011

"Clara wanted the wounded soldiers to receive proper care both on the battlefield and in the hospital."
>DK Biography: Clara Barton, A Photographic Story of a
>Life, page 60, Steven Krensky, DK Publishing, 2011

"When she finally returned home to Washington, Clara was by her own description, 'shoeless, gloveless, ragged, and blood-stained.' Whatever pride she might feel later in her actions, for the moment, she was consumed by "Desolation and pity and sympathy and weariness all blended.' By the Spring of 1863, she had recovered her strength."
>DK Biography: Clara Barton, A Photographic Story of a
>Life, page 61, Steven Krensky, DK Publishing, 2011.

Speaking of a nurse going out of her comfort zone to meet the needs of their patients and show them the comfort they needed, she went to the ultimate length to do this as did Gentle Annie, and Florence Nightingale.

This nurse was compassionate to the ump degree putting her patients needs far beyond that of her own needs and this is why she would eventually receive a Noble Peace Prize for being such a great nurse.

And when you see all this you wonder why it is that some of today's nurses complain they might have to go out of their comfort zone if they have to comfort their own patients who need their comfort and compassionate care. Like some of the qouters in this book have said, "Comfort has fallen out of line over the decades." And other qouters in this book stating, "Comfort has been relegated to end of life care" who also state that "comfort should be promoted for all stages of life and not just end of life care and at one time it was." What has happened to our nursing world? Where has compassion gone?

One book has it that they believe that Clara Barton was too shy to ask for a pair of gloves and that she was so timid it made her cry when her mother asked her about it because she was too shy to ask. I think this could very well be a possibility because I have this problem myself. But, I also have another problem that could be related to this. It may be that she was too shy to ask and too shy to answer her mother's question as they thought considering I do this myself. But, I think there's also a possibility she was too shy to even wear the gloves and it bothered her the whole time to wear them because it embarrassed her to have to wear them.

So when they were good and wore out and she had an excuse to say they were she may have been hoping to not ever have to wear a pair of gloves again if her mother thought that the gloves were worn out. If so, she probably just didn't want to say anything and didn't even ask if she could have new ones because she really didn't want them in the first place because it embarrassed her to death in the first place. It embarrasses me to wear a hat. I only wore one in the garden planting flowers because Bertha feared I'd get skin cancer from the sun. Otherwise, I wouldn't even wear them at all. Plus, they're uncomfortable anyway. But, notice something else. This book said she would suffer wrong first, but for others she would be fearless.

I have a feeling she probably wore gloves for working with patients but refrained from wearing them when she wasn't working with a patient in order to save herself the embarrassment. That definitely sounds like something I would do. I'm just like that. This helps me to bring out another point. Some nurses or doctors may say, "I don't think my nurses would be comfortable doing that" if I asked them to rub my head to calm me down through a needle stick or give me a hug, but this lady, Clara Barton would go out of her way to do things for others she would never do for herself.

Plus, on top of all that, as you are seeing from all the quotes from various nurses and doctors in this book as well as encyclopedias and medical school books, nurses are required to comfort their patients, and yes, that does mean rubbing their head to calm them down and holding their hand and giving them hugs and patting their shoulder etc. That's their job.

That's what they are, caregivers. And, the caregivers that take care of their patients in the doctor's offices and hospitals are supposed to take the place of the parent and treat their patients as if they were their own children. Why else do you think one of the qouters in this book said that nursing is a good foundation for learning to raise a family? And, why else do you think an electronic spelling thesaurus gadget is telling me that "to nurse" is to "act as a parent to" and the dictionary says "to nurse" is to "nurture" as do many encyclopedias and books?
This must be very enlightening seeing that some nurses today don't even realize it is part of their job to comfort their patients when they go to see them.

It is just as detrimental to a patient you take care of their need for physical comfort as it is to give them a bunch of shots and sew them up and fix up their wounds. Without physical comfort from the nurses caring for you what's the use in even going on if no one really cares?

In the book, "DK Biography, Clara Barton, A Photographic Story of a Life" by Steven Krensky we see Clara Barton make the following comment in her own memoirs:

"So far as our poor efforts can reach, they shall never lack a kindly hand or a sister's sympathy."
> DK Biography: Clara Barton, A Photographic Story of a Life, page 52, Steven Krensky, DK Publishing, 2011

In the Book, Clara Barton: Founder of the American Red Cross" it says this about Clara Barton. Clara's friend Susie got small pox and Clara took care of her and this was what was said about her:

"Mrs. White was grateful for all the help Clara gave. Clara seemed to know how to make her friend comfortable. She could "soothe" her when no one else could."
> Clara Barton: Founder of the American Red Cross, page 143, Augusta Stevenson, Aladdin Paperbacks, 1946 & 1962

"That child is a natural-born nurse," said Mrs. White. "I don't know how I'd manage without her. What a wonderful help."
> Clara Barton: Founder of the American Red Cross, page 143, Augusta Stevenson, Aladdin Paperbacks, 1946, & 1962

Now let me define the word soothe. The Funk & Wagnall's Standard Dictionary, 1985 defines it the following way.

Soothe – to restore to a quiet or normal state; calm, 2. to mitigate, soften, or relieve, as pain or grief, to have a calming or relieving effect
> Funk & Wagnall's Standard Desk Dictionary, Volume 2, N-Z, page 642, 1985

Notice it says to soothe is to restore to a quiet or normal state. It also says to soften or relieve in pain or grief and to have a calming or relieving effect on.

That's what nurses are there for, to soothe your patients, to return them to a quiet or normal state.

You want to soothe your patients and soften them and relieve them in pain and have a calming or relieving effect on them. When you comfort them with soothing words and lots of affection then this is what helps revive the patient to a normal state and make them feel cared for. You should do this even if they seem normal to you to begin with because you're hurting them emotionally when you don't. No matter what physical repairs you do for a patient from a technical standpoint, without comfort by affection and cheerful words they feel uncared for and everything you do is all for naught because then they go away a terrible mess from not having their needs met.

Once again, in the book "Clara Barton: Founder of the American Red Cross" you see "Clara hold up a soldier laying down, put her arm around him with one arm and give him a cup of water with the other hand at the same time."
> Clara Barton: Founder of the American Red Cross, page
> 181, Augusta Stevenson, Aladdin Paperbacks, 1946 & 1962

"Clara Barton was so well thought of by the soldiers that a large audience rose to its feet and a thousand voices called, "Mrs. Barton! Mrs. Barton!"
> Clara Barton: Founder of the American Red Cross, page
> 183, Augusta Stevenson, Aladdin Paperbacks, 1946 & 1962

"The lady bowed, smiled, and waved her hand. The applause went on and on."
> Clara Barton: Founder of the American Red Cross, page
> 183, Augusta Stevenson, Aladdin Paperbacks, 1946 & 1962

"When she finished speaking there was a long applause."
> Clara Barton: Founder of the American Red Cross, page
> 183, Augusta Stevenson, Aladdin Paperbacks, 1946, 1962

"They couldn't do enough to show how much they loved and respected her."
> Clara Barton: Founder of the American Red Cross, page
> 183, Augusta Stevenson, Aladdin Paperbacks, 1946 & 1962

Here's another word commonly used to describe how nurses are to be with their patients. They are to show empathy to their patients.

"Empathy is a social and emotional skill that helps us feel and understand the emotions, circumstances, intentions, thoughts, and needs of others, such that we can offer sensitive, perceptive, and appropriate communication and support."

> The Art of Empathy: A Complete Guide to Life's Most Essential Skill, page 3, Karla McLaren, Sounds True Incorporated, 2013

Since nurses are supposed to treat their patients like children, I'd like to point out what this book says about empathy toward babies. "Simply put, to develop empathy, a baby needs warm, nurturing attention from one or two reliable, central caregivers who touch, interact with, and respond attentively to his or her unique emotions and needs."

> The Art of Empathy: A Complete Guide to Life's Most Essential Skill, page 215, Karla McLaren, Sounds True Incorporated, 2013

"Babies, especially in their first year, need as much warm, emotive, and intimate human interaction as they can get" and that's how I am.

> The Art of Empathy: A complete Guide to Life's Most Essential Skill, page 215, Karla Mc Laren, Sounds True Incorporated, 2013

I'm autistic and I have childlike needs and these needs need to be met.

"Nurses offer patients "comfort" and advice".

> What Do They Do? Nurses, Jennifer Zeiger, page 8, Cherry Lane Publishing, 2010

"Sometimes patients need extra care. They might need special tests. Nurses help run the tests. They also prepare patients for operations. They also 'help people feel less scared' and help their pain go away."

>What Do They Do? Nurses, Jennifer Zeiger, page 8, Cherry Lane Publishing, 2010

On page 11 of the book, "What Do They DO? Nurses" you will see a friendly female nurse smiling and holding a girl patient's hand.

>What Do They Do? Nurses, page 11, Jennifer Zeiger, Cherry Lane Publishing, 2010

On page 15 of the book, "What Do They Do? Nurses" you will notice a nurse puts one hand behind the back of a male patient in a wheel chair and puts his other hand on his shoulder and looks at him and smiles.

>What Do They Do? Nurses, page 15, Jennifer Zeiger, Cherry Lane Publishing, 2010

The lady nurse on the cover of the book "What Do They Do? Nurses" is also smiling cheerfully at a girl patient as she takes her temperature.

>What Do They Do? Nurses, Jennifer Zeiger, Book Cover, July 2010

"Nursing is a profession that provides care to the sick, the injured and other people in need of medical assistance."

>World Book Encyclopedia Online, 2016

"Patients often get most of their direct health care through nurses. Nurses record patient medical histories and symptoms help perform medical tests, administer treatment and medications, operate medical machinery, and help with follow up care and rehabilitation. They also provide advice and "emotional support" to patients and their families.

>World Book Encyclopedia Online, 2016

"The Well Being of Patients is of first importance to nurses. RNs are taught to "recognize and understand patients' needs." They provide 'emotional support' as well as physical care, taking time to 'reassure worried patients and boost their morale'".
        World Book Encyclopedia Online, 2016

"Each type of patient has 'special needs' requiring nurses with 'specialized knowledge and training'".
        World Book Encyclopedia Online, 2016

"LPNs perform many patient care tasks."
        World Book Encyclopedia Online, 2016

Here are some more definitions I found from more current dictionaries about nursing.
Nurse – nourish, nurture; a person formally educated and trained in the care of the sick or infirm to tend to or minister to in sickness, infirmity, etc., encourage, abet, help, aid
        Stuart Berg Flexner & Lonore Crary Hawk, Random House Unabridged Dictionary, 2nd Edition, page 1331, Random House Inc., 1993

Nurture – tenderness and solicitude in training in mind and manners
        Stuart Berg Flexner & Lonore Crary Hawk, Random House Unabridged Dictionary, page 1331, 2nd Edition, Random House Inc., 1993

Nurse- a person educated and trained to care for the sick or "disabled", one that nurtures or fosters, to manage or guide carefully, look after with care, foster, nurture
        The American Heritage High School Dictionary, 3rd Edition, page 937, Houghton Mifflin, 1997

Caregiver – a person who assists a sick or "disabled" person who "attends to the needs of a child or dependent adult"
        The American Heritage High School Dictionary, 3rd Edition, page 212,
        Houghton Mifflin, 1997

Care – to have an inclination, fondness, liking, or affection, to feel concerned about; to watch over; be responsible for; a state of mind in which one is troubled; worry, anxiety, or concern
>Stuart Berg Flexner & Lonore Crary, Random House Unabridged Dictionary, Page 314, 315, 2nd Edition, 1993

Caregiver – a person who takes care of someone who is sick or "disabled"
>Stuart Berg Flexner & Lonore Crary, Random House Unabridged Dictionary, 2nd Edition, page 315, 1993

Nurture – support or encourage, foster
>Stuart Berg Flexner & Lonore Crary, Random House Unabridged Dictionary, 2nd Edition, page 1332, 1993

Tender – soft or delicate; delicate, soft or gentle: The tender touch of her hand, easily moved to sympathy or compassion, kind, a tender heart, affectionate or loving; sentimental or amendatory; a tender glance, considerate, or careful.
>Random House Unabridged Dictionary, 2nd Edition, page 1953, 1993

Loving – feeling or showing love; warmly affectionate; loving glances
>Stuart Berg Flexner & Lonore Crary, Random House Unabridged Dictionary,
>2nd Edition, pages 1139, 1140, 1993

"In a small book simply entitled 'On Caring" Milton Mayeroff (1972) lists eight major ingredients as necessary for caring. He describes these specifically in the context of a 'parent caring for a child', a teacher for a pupil, a psychotherapist for a patient, or a husband for his wife. Nurses are rarely in such a close or extended relationship with patients, but Mayeroff's concern is to show there is a pattern in helping others grow, which is what nurses generally do. Nurses do not necessarily help people to grow up, but they certainly help them grow in understanding of their illness and having to cope with it."

Ethics in Nursing: The Caring Relationship, Veronica
Tschudin, page 5, Butterworth – Heinemann, 1986, 1992;
Elsevier Limited, 2003

"In caring we need to know many things: 'who the other is', 'what
the person's needs are', and 'what helps the other'." We know that
some things work explicitly and others inexplicitly. One important
reason perhaps for our failure to realize how much knowing there
is in caring is our habit sometimes of restraining knowledge
arbitrarily to what can be verbalized." (Mayeroff 1972, page 10)

Ethics In Nursing: The Caring Relationship, page 5,
Veronica Tschudin, 2003

"Patricia Munhall (1993) described congently that nurses also need
to learn how to 'unknow' in order to be authentically present for
patients. This is not easy. However, unknowing – a kind of
'receptivity' or 'humility' – it is essential if we want to hear the
other person and learn what the other person is about."

Ethics in Nursing: The Caring Relationship, page 5,
Veronica, Tschudin, 2003

"Knowledge is conveyed both verbally and nonverbally."

Ethics in Nursing: The Caring Relationship, page 5,
Veronica Tschudin, 2003

"We do not wait passively for something to happen. We give it
our full attention. When we care, we have patience with people
and proceed at their pace. That can be frustrating, but it is vital if
real caring is to take place."

Ethics in Nursing: The Caring Relationship, page 6,
Veronica Tschudin, 2003

"Honesty – this is a positive, often active confrontation between
ourselves and the other. 'We need to be able to see the other as
that person is and not what we would like that individual to be."

Ethics in Nursing: The Caring Relationship, page 6,
Veronica Tschudin, 2003

"Trust involves an appreciation of the other, of that person's independent existence. It also means we have confidence in our ability to help. We must also trust the other and this includes letting go or leaping into the unknown."
> Ethics in Nursing: The Caring Relationship, page 6,
> Veronica Tschudin, 2003

"When we are open to each person and situation, then each relationship is unique. We cannot simply do what we did in the last case; we have to learn all the time. This learning means constant restarting, or 'unknowing'. Humility sees others as existing for themselves, not as a means of self – fulfillment. Caring teaches us our true 'limitations and strengths'. We must accept both with humility."
> Ethics in Nursing: The Caring Relationship, Veronica
> Tschudin, 2003

"Hope is not wishful thinking, but an expression of the fullness of the present alive with a sense of the possible. The process of caring is possible only because hope is always present."
> Ethics in Nursing: The Caring Relationship, page 6,
> Veronica Tschudin, 2003

"In caring and growing we go into the unknown: caring can only be experienced, and the quality of that experience is what matters."
> Ethics in Nursing: The Caring Relationship, pages 7, 8,
> Veronica Tschudin, 2003

"Care is the basic element of being a person. In caring a man lives the meaning of his own life. When we do not care, we lose our 'being' and caring is the way back into being." (Roach 1992, page 58)
> Ethics in Nursing, The Caring Relationship, page 8
> Veronica Tschudin, 2003

"Compassion may be defined as a way of living born out of the awareness to all living creatures." (Roach 1992, page 58)
> Ethics in Nursing: The Caring Relationship, page 8,
> Veronica Tschudin, 2003

"Compassion asks us to go where it hurts, to enter into places of pain, to share in brokenness, fear confusion, and anguish. Compassion challenges us to cry out with those in misery, mourn with those who are lonely, to weep with those in tears."

>Ethics in Nursing: The Caring Relationship, page 8,
>Veronica Tschudin, 2003

That's what I want in a nurse, someone I can cry on when I am in distress and be able to receive their comfort. I also need hugs (be able to put my right ear on their cheek), and them to rub the top of my head to calm me down and hold my hand through needle sticks.

"Compassion requires us to be weak with the weak, vulnerable with the vulnerable, and powerless with the powerless. Compassion means full immersion in the condition of being human."

>Ethics in Nursing: The Caring Relationship, page 8,
>Veronica Tschudin, 2003

"Nurses care when they are present with another with a closeness that evokes compassion. Hence the caring nurse is focused on the 'other' that the 'other's' welfare is paramount."

>Ethics in Nursing: The Caring Relationship, page 9,
>Veronica Tschudin, 2003

"Compassion is a complex aspect of caring. It demands above all knowledge of one's self and one's values."

>Ethics in Nursing: The Caring Relationship, page 10,
>Veronica Tschudin, 2003

"Compassion is more specific than caring. Compassion questions, brings to closure, and defends others. Caring calls for the caring; compassion is there when it hurts. Caring can be professional, but compassion has to be experienced."

>Ethics in Nursing: The Caring Relationship, page 10,
>Veronica Tschudin, 2003

"Caring can be learnt, but compassion comes out of the experience of one having been hurt and having been shown compassion. We do not respond to compassion out of a sense of duty but out of a sense of solidarity."
> Ethics in Nursing: The Caring Relationship, page 10, Veronica Tschudin, 2003

"Competence is a state of having the knowledge, judgment, skills, energy, experience, and motivation required to respond adequately to the demands of one's professional responsibilities. (Roach, 1991, page 161)
> Ethics in Nursing: The Caring Relationship, page 10, Veronica Tschudin, 2003

"Caring does demand competence, but competence with a human face. Care has to be appropriate, adequate, and practiced with respect considering the 'needs of those who are the recipient."
> Ethics in Nursing: The Caring Relationship, Veronica Tschudin, page 11, 2003

"Confidence is defined as quality that fosters trusting relationships. Most nurses would agree that at the basis of caring lies a trusting relationship. Confidence is reciprocal; both parties in a relationship need to trust each other."
> Ethics in Nursing: The Caring Relationship, Veronica Tschudin, page 11, 2003

"Conscience can be defined as a state of moral awareness; a compass directing one's behavior according to the moral fitness of things. Conscience is the call of care and manifests itself as care."
> Ethics in Nursing: The Caring Relationship, page 12, Veronica Tschudin, 2003

"Commitment is a complex effective response characterized by a convergence between one's desires and one's obligations, and by a deliberate choice to act in accordance with them. (Roach, 1992, page 65)
> Ethics in Nursing: The Caring Relationship, Veronica Tschudin, page 12, Butterworth-Heinemann, 2002; Elseiner Limited, 2003

Nurses should be committed to meeting their patients' needs. "Care giving is something practical, something done to someone by someone."
> Ethics in Nursing: The Caring Relationship, Veronica Tschudin, page 14, Butterworth – Heinemann, 2002; Elseiner Limited, 2003

"Caring involves for the caregiver first of all a 'feeling with the other.'
Empathy is 'suffering in'. How would I feel in that position?"
> Ethics in Nursing: The Caring Relationship, Veronica Tschudin, page 14, Butterworth – Heinemann, 2002; Elseiner Limited, 2003

This is how nurses should be with their patients.

"Lisa H. Newton in her defense of the traditional role of the nurse appeals to an argument based on the patient's needs. Because a patient may not be able to take care of himself Newton points out, 'his entire self concept of an independent human being may be threatened'…He needs 'comfort', 'reassurance', 'someone to talk to', the person he really needs, who would be taking care of all these problems is his mother, and 'the first job of the nurse is to be a mother surrogate.'"
> Caring: Nurses, Women, and Ethics, Helga Kuhse, page 58, Blackwell Publishers, 1997

"In the interactions of nurses with clients, a key energetic is 'presence', a mutual 'being with' between nurse and client. True presence often leaves nurses feeling vulnerable and in a state of 'not knowing'.

> Caring: The Compassionate Healer, Deloris A. Gout, page 56, 1991 Madeline M. Leininger, Center for Human Caring, National League of National Nursing Press, New York, Publication Number 15-2401, 1991

"Nurses are frequently challenged to energetically 'stay present' and face the unknown and unknowable with their clients. The discomfort of 'not knowing' raises a need in us to understand transpersonal energetics lest they be perceived as dangerous. Otherwise, in order to protect ourselves we might opt to contract our consciousness, limiting the extent to which we are willing to be fully present to the client. This may be understood as self-protection from the energetic occupational hazards of nursing and may be conscious or unconscious on the part of the nurse."

> Caring: The Compassionate Healer, Deloris A. Gout, page 56, 1991, Madeline M. Leininger, Center for Human Caring, National League of Nursing Press, New York, Publication Number 15-2401, 1991

"This author's background in the study, practice and teaching of 'therapeutic touch' provides a basis for addressing the energetic phenomena involved here."

> Caring: The Compassionate Healer, Deloris A. Gout, page 56, 1991, Madeline M. Leininger, Center for Human Caring, National League of Nursing Press, New York, Publication Number 15-2401, 1991

"An image present by Dr. Janet Quinn (1982) in a class she taught on Therapeutic Touch comes to mind. Dr. Quinn said as nurses walk down the corridor of the hospital, or any setting in which they provide care, they can almost feel the needs of the clients reaching out to them, as though they are there with fishing rods and reels, casting out as nurses go by and hooking them energetically. How do nurses deal with this?" she asked.

"An excellent question", she said. The 'needs' that represent the hook clients use to snag nurses with are 'in fact the same reason nurses are there; to meet the clients needs which are their call for nursing."

> Caring: The Compassionate Healer, pages 56, 57, 1991, Madeline M. Leininger, Center for Human Caring, National League of Nursing Press, New York, Publication Number 15-2401, 1991

With me I always want a hug. If you see me longingly looking at you or reaching out for you or even trying to catch up with you, all I want is a hug. I need to be able to put my right ear on your cheek because I have a sensory issue in my right ear that can only be relieved by pressing it on the cheek of the people I like. This is especially needful when I am scared, but I also need this even if I am not scared because it puts me at chaos not to be able to and traumatizes me as a result when I am refused a hug. I may also be trying to get your attention to come comfort me if I think I am about to get stuck with a needle because I need you to rub the top of my head and hold my hand through a needle stick when another nurse sticks me with a needle, and both the nurse sticking me and the one comforting me need to be chipper acting, cheery female nurses with a motherly personality.

"Often these needs present as fear and pain, sadness, anguish, loss, grief, or anger, anxiety, and frustration."

> Caring: The Compassionate Healer, page 57, Madeline M. Leininger, Center for Human Caring, National League of Nursing Press, New York, Publication Number 15-2401, 1991

It can be this way with me too, usually "fear", "pain", and "anxiety", or "frustration."

"Of course, nurses also experience peace, hope, love, surrender, and other poignant moments of human beauty with clients. However, these moments are not as threatening to us as the moments listed initially are."

> Caring: The Compassionate Healer, page 57, Madeline M. Leininger, Center for Human Caring, National League of Nursing Press, New York, Publication Number 15-2401, 1991

When you go in thinking, hey, I need to be willing to touch these people (your patients) and be willing to give them hugs and shoulder pats and head rubs, etc. because I am a nurse and I need to tend to their needs they have and be like a mother to them it all works out better in the end and you feel safer with them and they feel safer with you.

"If we envision the process of being with the client as energetic engagement, the nature of the threat, the reality of the danger becomes clear. As nurses openly engage with clients, they experience energetic absorption of their client's fear and pain and resonate with their client's frustration and anger."

> Caring: The Compassionate Healer, page 57, Madeline M. Leininger, Center for Human Caring, National League of Nursing Press, New York, Publication Number 15-2401, 1991

"However, these energetics only represent dangers in so far as nurse are unconscious of them, or unprepared to respond in a way that sustains the nurse's capacity to simultaneously "nurture the client" and them self."

> Caring: The Compassionate Healer, page 57, Madeline M. Leininger, Center for Human Caring, National League of Nursing Press, New York, Publication Number 15-2401, 1991

"Lack of self renewal skills and a tendency to empathize with emotional hurt of clients may lead to a tendency for nurses to energetically withdraw. This may take the form of focusing on the tasks and doing rather than 'being with", as the primary nursing activity with clients."

> Caring: The Compassionate Healer, page 57, Madeline M. Leininger, Center for Human Caring, National League of Nursing Press, New York, Publication Number 15-2401, 1991

"This is antithetical to the caring role that is the heart of nursing. It undercuts nurse's capacity to be compassionate and surely minimizes the therapeutic value of the nursing interaction for clients."

> Caring: The Compassionate Healer, page 57, Madeline M. Leininger, Center for Human Caring, National League of Nursing Press, New York, Publication Number 15-2401, 1991

Hopefully you realize this lady is talking about patients. She just keeps referring to them as clients.

"Gadov (1989) reflects that this is not only something that nurses do in the perceived threatening moments presented here, but is something nurses learn early in their careers."

> Caring: The Compassionate Healer, page 57, Madeline Leininger, Center for Human Caring, National League of Nursing Press, New York, Publication Number 15-2401, 1991

"It is easier for nurses to regard clients as objects and take a disembodied view to 'avoid embarrassing themselves and the patients to expedite awkward procedures and to avoid feeling pain when inflicting pain on patients'."

> Caring: The Compassionate Healer, page 57, Madeline Leininger, Center for Human Caring, National League of Nursing Press, New York, Publication Number 15-2401, 1991

I think what she means is, when you give your patient a shot, or a blood test, or an IV, or insert tubes or catheters in your patients or fix their wounds and you don't want to show them how you truly feel about having to do this to them because it embarrasses you to have to admit it bothers you to hurt them. But, you still need to comfort them and show compassion no matter how you feel. You're hurting their feelings when you don't in the process, and you're for sure hurting my feelings when you do this.

Here is a comment I found about Rehabilitative Nurses in a College Text Book on Rehabilitative Nursing:

"Is it the nurse that maintains an orderly unit with policies and procedures which ensure a comfortable and secure environment for the patient? The Nurse may never quite realize the security represented by this visit to the patient who has waited hours to have someone enter the room. Patients learn quickly when a shift starts, who is on and who is off, when a nurse is not feeling well, and when a nurse is feeling great. If there is a bit of warmth, a caring response that the patient can elicit, the patient will become an expert at obtaining it and will learn quickly to expect it – perhaps because the need is so desperate. Within a matter of hours, the patients become dependent on an unfamiliar structure and on unknown faces who use an unfamiliar medical language. They do not know if something will cause pain or not, or whether they will be heard or responded to when the need to be heard or responded to arises."

Comprehensive Rehabilitation Nursing, McGraw Hill, 1981, Nancy Martin, RN, MA; Nancye B. Holt, RN, MS; Dorothy Hicks, RN, MN, pages 6 & 7

"In the hospital environment, patients for the most part find it difficult to decide crucial issues of their own well-being. Burdened by the disintegrative and anxiety-provoking aspects of their illnesses, they do not know how to deal with procedures personally, particularly when they have no idea at the significance of the procedures. They are, or feel they are at the mercy of the medical staff, the nursing staff, and the policies and procedures set by administration. Their apprehension inevitably inhibits trust and confidence in the hospital and staff. And the nursing department must deal with this lack of trust every hour, 24 hours a day, and 168 hours a week."

> Comprehensive Rehabilitation Nursing, McGraw Hill, 1981, Nancy Martin, RN, MA; Nancye B. Holt, RN, MS; Dorothy Hicks, RN, MN, pages 6 & 7

"Patients expect the hospital and its staff to render attentive, quality care, and they pay handsomely for that care. Professionals in the hospital environment should exercise the responsibilities and obligations appropriately expected by patients-the responsibilities professionals have been trained for and are paid for.

> Comprehensive Rehabilitation Nursing, McGraw Hill, 1981, Nancy Martin, RN, MA; Nancye B. Holt, RN, MS; Dorothy Hicks, RN, MN, page 7

"If nurses allow themselves to be as human as patients, particularly when dealing with patients, and cannot set aside those burdensome human qualities which interfere, then possibly they have been trained for the wrong profession. It is the rehabilitation nurse who assists so greatly in restoring the disabled person."

> Comprehensive Rehabilitation Nursing, McGraw Hill, 1981, Nancy Martin, RN, MA; Nancye B. Holt, RN, MS; Dorothy Hicks, RN, MN, page 7

This is the way this book is saying that Rehabilitative nurses need to be with their patients, but as you will see throughout my book, this is also the way all nurses in all hospitals and doctors offices need to be with their patients in every department they work in.

"Gadov (1989) observes that nurses learn to regard their own bodies as objects, thereby becoming 'disembodied caregivers', 'disassociating from their own bodies' in avoidance of experiencing that patient's pain."

> Caring: The Compassionate Healer, page 57, Madeline Leininger, Center for Human Caring, National League of Nursing Press, New York, Publication Number 15-2401, 1991

I feel like you guys think I am a car you're fixing when you do this and it hurts my feelings drastically. The past couple of years I've ran into a lot of nurses that refuse to hug me or comfort me through a needle stick because they think I am somehow in the wrong and they think it is not in their job description to do so, when in fact it is in your job description. You may have not been told you have to hug patients or comfort them through needle sticks when you were hired, but both your school books in nursing and your nurse exam say that you are required to comfort your patients. I have seen this proven several times over in a college textbook of nursing I found just recently.

Here is a quote in "Caring-The Compassionate Healer" I found regarding nurses that disassemble themselves from their patients.

"She further suggests that in order to provide care in the intersubjective framework, nurses must be willing to re-embody, which again raises the issue of vulnerability and safety. Courage and devotion are necessary for nurses to consciously make the choice to be fully present and energetically open in a compassionate way that facilitates wholeness for clients."

> Caring: The Compassionate Healer, page 57, Madeline Leininger, Center for Human Caring, National League of Nursing Press, New York, Publication Number 15-2401, 1991

"In this regard, Therapeutic Touch offers nurses a mode of clinical intervention as well as personal energy management knowledge and skills."

> Caring: The Compassionate Nurse, The Compassionate Healer, page 57, Madeline Leininger, Center for Human Caring, National League of Nursing Press, New York, Publication 15-2401, 1991

"The nurses' capacity to engage in conscious caring from an energetic perspective then becomes part of his or her lived experience of nursing, and ongoing self study."

> Caring: The Compassionate Nurse, The Compassionate Healer, page 57, Madeline Leininger, Center for Human Caring, National League of Nursing Press, New York, Publication 15-2401, 1991

I actually have the same "sick sense" tendency you all have about patients as a nurse, but instead of being driven away from it; I am actually drawn to it. I would do for anyone what I am asking you to do for me and this is what I need. One time when I was a teenager, a youth group from my church went to visit some residents at a nursing home. When I walked in the door I heard this guy moaning and I was immediately saddened and drug down and depressed by it. I felt like I could feel his pain and I wished there was something I could do about it but felt horrible because I felt like there wasn't anything I can do. When I come to you like this, I feel like you want to run the other way, but when I ran into these people I was drawn by them instead of being turned away.

I was actually a nurse aide at an Alzheimer's Center and then a nursing home back in 1996 and I was this way with all the patients I ever worked with. I was so drawn to the patients I was to take care of to the point that the other nurse aide's told me I wasn't assertive enough and that I let the other patients drag me down too much. That's just the way I am.

Have you ever heard the phrase "Do unto others what you would have them do unto you?"

I feel like I am getting the raw end of the deal because I did all this for my patients but yet when I'm the patient I get nurses sometimes that say, "It's not in my job description to comfort you or give you a hug."

Actually, as you can obviously see, it really is in your job description. Your employer may not have told you when they hired you that you needed to comfort your patients when they came to you and you were their nurse, but your classes you took and your nurse exam you took to get your nurse's license did say it was in your job description, so that being kept in mind, the employer already assumed in most cases that you knew that was "a given" already without them even telling you that you were supposed to do all this because you were already supposed to know all this from your own schooling before you even became a nurse. Sometimes I wonder if they even know. I've ran into a few of them that didn't. Some of you that see me as a needy person are already drawn to me when I act this way toward you, but other nurses who cannot see I am needy and think I look normal to them shrug away or walk away because they think what I am asking is not proper to them when in fact it is their job as a nurse to act as my "mother surrogate" which is what I need. It hurts my feelings tremendously when you do shrug away or walk away or act mad when I am asking you for your comfort or for a hug (put my right ear on your cheek). It's so hard to get you to see my needs are genuine as normal as I look. I am actually an Ex-Special Ed student but I have been normalized to such a point that you can't even see it. I'm really one of them and I still have the same childlike needs now that I had back then. These needs never went away and they will never go away. I will always need them met for the rest of my life. I am disabled and this is what I need. I am autistic. There are some nurses who see my needs that only meet them because of this knowledge. Technically, you are already required to do this for every patient, whether they are disabled or not, but especially me because I am disabled and I need your comfort. It tears me apart when you don't meet my needs and refuse to give me a hug (let me put my right ear on your cheek).

It also tears me apart when you refuse to rub my head to calm me down and hold my hand through an IV stick, blood test, shot, biopsy, or anything else that is sharp that both hurts me and scares me. That's what you're there for. You're supposed to treat me as a child and comfort me like a mother comforts her child or baby and be a mother to me. I need all of you to be like mommies and buddies to me. I know this sounds strange to you but this is what you are there for and I have childlike needs and need you to meet my needs. And, they are genuine needs. Not meeting these needs actually traumatizes me. One of the people I quoted apparently stated this does this to other people who are as vulnerable as I am. Please see to it that you meet my needs for hugs and comfort. I'm autistic and I crave touch and require a lot of affection. I always have and always will require a lot of affection. It's the way I am because of my autism. Please try to understand. I really need this.

"Promoting a client's psychosocial integrity is not just for the mental health client, but for 'all' clients."
> Kaplan NCLEX-RN 2014-2015 – Strategies, Practice, and Review with Practice Test, page 186, Kaplan Inc., 2014

"Nurses, not families, are responsible for 'all' the hands on nursing care for clients in the hospital."
> Kaplan NCLEX-RN 2014-2015 – Strategies, Practice, and Review with Practice Test, page 186, Kaplan Inc., 2014

"A patient removed from his usual setting is removed from his usual support systems. When admitted to a hospital, he is experiencing illness while adapting to the environment and culture of the hospital. The abrupt change from a familiar to an unfamiliar residence, along with the stress associated with illness and loss of support system, may precipitate a type of cultural shock."
> Basic Nursing: A Psychophysiologic Approach, W.B. Saunders Company, 1979, Sorenson, Luckman, page 526

"The farther the hospital from the patient's home, the greater the loss of support, and, potentially, the greater the stress."
> Basic Nursing: A Psychophysiologic Approach, W.B. Saunders Company, 1979, Sorenson, Luckman, page 526

"In the hospital "culture" are many factors that threaten the self-concept of the patient. Fear, loneliness and anxiety, all common reactions to loss of health, need expression in order for healing to occur on the emotional level along with the physical level."

> Basic Nursing: A Psychophysiologic Approach, W.B. Saunders Company, 1979, Sorenson, Luckman, page 526

Finally, psychologic comfort may be disturbed by factors influencing stimulation of the patient's senses. In addition, thoughtful actions such as 'touching the patient', identifying time and place, describing outside environmental conditions, explaining care and treatment and listening to the patient may enhance the quality of care the patient perceives."

> Basic Nursing: A Psychophysiologic Approach, W.B. Saunders Company, 1979, Sorenson, Luckman, page 527

"Nurses care for the whole person, not just all illness. Their focus is on 'client needs'; that is how a client will respond to an illness."

> Kaplan Nursing, NCLEX-RN, 2014-2015, Strategies, Practice, and Review with Practice Test, page 455, Kaplan Inc., 2014

"Key Features of US-Style communication in nursing includes: conveying respect and 'warmth' making the client 'feeling accepted' and 'respected' as an individual 'regardless of his or her words, actions, or behaviors.'" This means the nurse: "accepts the 'dependency needs' of the client while encouraging, assisting, and supporting movement toward health and independence."

> Kaplan Nursing, NCLEX-RN, 2014-2015, Strategies, Practice, and Review with Practice Test, page 456, Kaplan Inc., 2014

"Certain forms of "touching" behaviors indicate "affection". For example, cheek patting, hand patting, and chucking under the chin are valued forms of affection in North America. The "laying on of hands" is a common expression indicating curative and comfort actions. This expression is often attributed to individuals in the healing professions such as religion, medicine, or 'nursing'. Tactile contacts vary considerably among individuals, families, and cultures. Some families have a great deal of tactile contact between all members of the family. Other families, even within the same culture have minimal contact. Appropriate forms of 'touch' can be helpful in 'reinforcing caring feelings' by the 'nurse'. The use of 'touch' alone often says much more than words for many patients such as those who are terminally ill or who are unable to speak."

> Fundamentals of Nursing: Concepts and Procedures, Barbara Kozier and Glenora Lea Erb, Addison-Wesley Publishing Company, 1979, page 407

"Disabled persons are entitled to have their 'special needs' taken into consideration at all stages of economic and social planning."

> Fundamentals of Nursing: Concepts and Procedures, Barbara Kozier and Glenora Lea Erb, Addison-Wesley Publishing Company, 1979, page 77, Declaration on the Rights of Disabled Persons, #8

I am autistic and this should apply to me.

"In the Declaration on the Rights of Disabled Persons adopted by the General Assembly of the United Nations in December 1975 thirteen points are made. This declaration includes the definition of disabled '…deficiency, either congenital or not, in his or her physical or mental capabilities.'"

> Fundamentals of Nursing: Concepts and Procedures, Barbara Kozier and Glenora Lea Erb, Addison-Wesley Publishing Company, 1979, page 76, Rights of Special Groups

The American Hospital Association (AHA) approved a Patient's Bill of Rights in 1973; the United Nations adopted the Declaration of the Rights of Disabled Persons in December, 1975. Bills are being passed that provide for the rights of patients in some states and provinces. Since the publication of the AHA Bill, a number of other rights statements have been made public, notably for the handicapped, the dying, the retarded and the elderly."

> Fundamentals of Nursing: Concepts and Procedures, Barbara Kozier and Glenora Lea Erb, Addison-Wesley Publishing Company, 1979, page 76, Rights of Special Groups

So, these nurses are supposed to meet my "special needs" because I am disabled and I do have special needs.

"Nurses are repeatedly faced with divided responsibility. On the one hand, the nurse is frequently an employee responsible to a hospital or health agency. On the other hand, the nurse is a professional person responsible to the professional ethics of an association and the standards of the profession. Last, the nurse is responsible to and for patients and is taught to respond to their needs in a therapeutic manner."

> Fundamentals of Nursing: Concepts and Procedures, Barbara Kozier and Glenora Lea Erb, Addison-Wesley Publishing Company, 1979, page 66

"The need for love is so basic that it has been described as the bony structure of man's whole emotional life (Caprio 1965:16). So much has been written on the subject of love by philosophers, poets, novelists, and behavioral scientists that the meaning of love is not always clear. To define love is difficult. There are many kinds of love, such as 'mother love', romantic love, love between friends and family members and love of God.

Perhaps it is enough to understand that love is accomplished with the heart and not the mind, that love is a feeling-an acting response rather than an intellectual process. Love is also a strong positive feeling that is not possessive. Some characteristics of love are outlined as follows:

1. Love is not only a subjective feeling that a person has (an emotion) but also a series of acts by which one person conveys to another the feeling that someone is deeply involved and profoundly interested in the person and the person's welfare.
2. Love is unconditional; it makes no bargains but conveys that one person is concerned for another person, that someone is there to give support and to contribute to the other's development as best as possible because the one values the other for what he is and as he is.
3. Love is supportive; it conveys to the other that you will always be present when the person most needs you, that you will neither condemn nor condone but that you will be there to offer your sympathy and understanding. Whatever the other needs as a human being she shall have. It is tolerant but not dependent (Montague 1974:15)

Fundamentals of Nursing: Concepts and Procedures, Barbara Kozier and Glenora Lea Erb, Addison-Wesley Publishing Company, 1979, page 106, The Need for Love and Affection, Love and Belonging Needs

"The need for love is met in many ways. In some situations, nurses can become the "surrogate parents" for young children who are in the hospital by supplying them with the "affection" and the "physical closeness" they need. With adults and elderly people the role of the nurse is less concrete. However, "in all instances" and interest in the welfare of people and a caring and supportive attitude need to be communicated. These can be conveyed in many ways: by 'touching', by 'staying with a patient when a patient is frightened', and by listening and communicating in a friendly manner."

Fundamentals of Nursing: Concepts and Procedures, Barbara Kozier and Glenora Lea Erb, Addison-Wesley Publishing Company, 1979, page 106, The Need for Love and Affection, Love and Belonging Needs

"A nurse can help build trust and security with a patient by (a) being a real person herself (genuineness); (b) "caring warmly" for the patient (nonpossessive warmth); and (c) attempting to understand him accurately (accurate empathy).
> Basic Nursing: A Psychophysiologic Approach, W.B.
> Saunders Company, 1979, Sorenson, Luckman, page 39

"Nurses are responsible for 'meeting the needs' of clients whose care involves technical equipment."
> Kaplan Nursing, Kaplan NCLEX-RN, 2014-2015,
> Strategies, Practice, and Review, page 456, Kaplan Inc.,
> 2014

"Rehabilitation begins when a patient first comes in contact with a health professional. It is not the final stage of treatment. On the contrary, rehabilitation is the underlying theme of all nursing and medical care.
> Basic Nursing: A Psychophysiologic Approach, W.B.
> Saunders Company, 1979, Sorenson, Luckman, page 241

"Rehabilitation involves assessment of the patient's physical and psychosocial needs and abilities. Both short-term and long-term assessments are necessary. A skillful nurse consistently evaluates the care she gives in relation to the previously identified, individualized patient's needs and goals."
> Basic Nursing: A Psychophysiologic Approach, W.B.
> Saunders Company, 1979, Sorenson, Luckman, page 241

"Creating a therapeutic environment means providing circumstances within which a person can feel comfortable and can work toward health when this is possible. This involves consideration of 'physical comfort' and 'psychological comfort'."
> Basic Nursing: A Psychophysiologic Approach, W.B.
> Saunders Company, 1979, Sorenson, Luckman, page 30

"While a nurse can get great satisfaction from her work, the helpful nurse does not allow her personal needs to take precedence over the needs of the patient. The helpful nurse is a "real person" within the nurse-patient relationship. However, the focus of the interactions is directed toward "patient need".

> Basic Nursing: A Psychophysiologic Approach, W.B. Saunders Company, 1979, Sorenson, Luckman, page 26

If you guys ever do a CT or MRI on me that require IV contrast, I'm sorry but you're going to have to give me hugs and rub my head to calm me down and hold my hand through the IV stick to comfort me or I'm not sticking around. IVs are too excruciating for me to be made to handle awake because being stuck with an IV feels like being stabbed with a butcher knife. I can't be expected to just handle it like everybody else because the pain is too excruciating for me and is too incredible a thing for me to handle without your comfort. Please don't make me do this.

I have to be comforted through my IVs and I've got to be able to have my hugs (be able to put my right ear on your cheek), especially in scary situations like these. I also need to be able to put Lidocaine/Prilocaine 2.5% cream on the site of the stick before you even stick me in the arm or anywhere else. And, if any of you get the bright idea to put a catheter in me for any reason I need to be put completely to sleep before you do. If I should go to your hospital for some reason and for some reason I started having trouble going to the bathroom something tremendous again, which would not be unusual, I can't just let you stand back and say, "Well, I guess we're going to have to put a catheter in him, get the catheter out and let's do this." The pain is so excruciating for me to have a catheter put in it's like having a sword being run through me. This is way too excruciating for me and way to incredible for me to handle. If you ever put a catheter in me, I need to be put to sleep first before you stick one in me. One time a doctor in Branson tried to make me do one of those Urethrogram cystoscopies a wake and barely got in the tip and I screamed like wildfire. I was in so much pain that I kicked the stirrups off the bed it was so excruciating. I wasn't even mad.

It was actually a reflex from reacting to the severity of the excruciating pain I was in, but they stopped the test after I did this and screamed both and the nurse told my wife, "I'll give him one more chance if he wants to try again in a week, otherwise we're not doing it again. He needs to learn to behave himself!"

I also went for a Urodynamics test at a Urologist's office in Arkansas one place and the APN nurse refused to put me to sleep. I almost backed out but the Urologist I went to insisted I have one before he did the TUIP surgery he was originally going to do because another Urologist swayed his opinion about what was wrong with me. When I went in for the test, I begged the female nurse assistant to the APN to comfort me but she refused to comfort me. Then, the APN began to insert the catheter and I went ballistic, screaming in excruciating pain and shaking and moaning in between. The female nurse assistant, who originally thought I was just trying to get inappropriate attention by asking her to comfort me, suddenly got shook up after I continued to be in pain and panic half way through the insertion.
She suddenly put her hand on my shoulder and started rubbing it and saying, "Its okay. Its okay. We're half way there, okay. Just please, try to make it okay. We're almost there, just a little bit longer." The girl was trembling in fear at how horrible the pain was I was experiencing from the catheter and almost lost it. The APN said, "I'm sorry! I'm taking it out! I'm hurting him too much!" The girl looked at me with severe disappointment about to cry and trying to hold back the tears and said, "I'm sorry! I didn't know! I'm so sorry!" The APN just acted angry and the female nurse assistant that assisted her acted like she was about to ball it was so bad, apologizing all over the place to me for not understanding me. It was not a good experience at all, and the girl was sorry she didn't just listen to me and comfort me through the procedure from the start. When I left, I was having sharp pains in the urethra and started bleeding. We rushed to my family doctor nearly 100 miles away and he had to give me AZO standard for bladder spasms to make the sharp pains go away and help stop the bleeding. It was horrible. It is not a good idea to make me do a catheter insertion awake. Please don't try it.

I did get another Urodynamics test by a different Urologist who was nicer a year later who said I was holding 600 to 900 ml of urine in my bladder and that was dangerous and that my bladder was shutting down. He shot Lidocaine into the area he inserted the catheter but the pain was still excruciating beyond end. That guy had a nurse at my bed from head to toe on both sides of the bed and had me trapped in the bed so I couldn't get away. They barely got me through it. They almost failed themselves. I don't know how they got by with getting me through it because no one else could. That same Urologist promised to never make me do a test awake again and put me to sleep for all my Cystoscopies he did on me from there on out.

The pain is so excruciating to me that the same goes for heart catheters, as well as urinary catheters, or any tubes of any kind.

A shot and a blood test feel like a steak knife, an IV feels like being stabbed with a butcher knife, and a catheter feels like a sword being run through me.

I don't think I can even handle you putting a tube down my throat awake for an EGD or Laryngoscopy, etc. It's just way too incredible for me to handle. I was asleep for my heart cath test. I would not chance making me do it awake. There's no telling what might go wrong. The pain is too excruciating, and I have a gag reflex.

Please, have mercy on me and meet my needs the way I am asking you to meet my needs.

And, remember, male doctors and male nurses, and male techs tortured me as a child. Serious trended female nurses also tortured me in childhood and adulthood.

Please do not give me either of these.

I need you to give me all female staff only. I need chipper acting, cheery female nurses with motherly personalities and cheery ones only to do all the sticks and insertions and the comforting, and especially the comforting part.

They are the ones I am comfortable with, and when they comfort me the way I ask them to with hugs and physical affection (hugs: put my right ear on their cheek, and physical affection: rub my head to calm me down and hold my hand to help me through needle sticks) and cheer me up with kind words and act sweetly to me like mommies and buddies to me, this is what works for me and this is what I need.

This is what Kaplan Nursing says about the nursing process and psychosocial integrity:

"You utilize the nursing process cases, diagnose, plan, implement, and evaluate to promote a client's psychosocial integrity by conveying 'understanding', 'sensitivity', and 'compassion' to a client who is experiencing stress, illness, or crisis."

>Kaplan Nursing, NCLEX-RN 2014-2015, page 186,
>Strategies and Practice and Review with Practice Test,
>Kaplan, Inc., 2014

"Nurses provide care for clients who constantly interact with their environment. 'Clients may have unmet needs', be unable to take care for themselves or be unable to adapt to the environment due to health problems. 'You' provide therapeutic care so clients can adapt to their environment."

>Kaplan NCLEX-RN, Kaplin Nursing, page 186, Strategies,
>Practice, and Review With Practice Test, Kaplin, Inc., 2014

"You need to identify clients at risk for 'sensory perceptual' alterations so you can initiate prevention measures."

>Kaplan NCLEX-RN, Kaplin Nursing, page 186, Strategies,
>Practice, and Review With Practice Test, Kaplin, Inc., 2014

"Examples of Clients at Risk include those who are confined in a non-stimulating environment, have impaired vision or hearing, have mobility restrictions, have emotional disorders, have limited social contact, are actively ill, are closely monitored (such as in the ICU), have decreased cognitive ability (as in a head injury), or are experiencing pain or discomfort."
> Kaplin NCLEX-RN, Kaplin Nursing, page 183, Strategies, Practice, and Review With Practice Test, Kaplan Inc., 2014

"When dealing with such a client you should organize nursing care to reduce unessential stimuli; orient the Client to person, place, and time during every contact, and explain nursing care."
> Kaplin NCLEX-RN, Kaplin Nursing, page 183, Strategies, Practice, and Review With Practice Test, Kaplan Inc., 2014

Autistic people have sensory issues and these needs need met when they have them.

"You should also listen attentively, provide an atmosphere of 'warmth' and trust, provide functional information as needed, and encourage clients to participate in the plan of care, promote safety and security and public education."
> Kaplan Nursing, Kaplan NCLEX-RN 2014-2015, Strategies, Practice and Review With Practice Test, page 484, Kaplan Inc., 2014

"In summary, the nurse who is alert to the patient's need for psychologic comfort will use a variety of creative ways to incorporate such measures into her caring ministry."
> Basic Nursing: A Psychophysiologic Approach, W.B. Saunders Company, 1979, Sorenson, Luckman, page 527

"Instrumental and expressive functions complement each other. No matter how efficiently a nurse performs instrumental tasks, their effectiveness will be reduced if she does not practice expressive roles in a sensitive and caring way."
> Basic Nursing: A Psychophysiologic Approach, W.B. Saunders Company, 1979, Sorenson, Luckman, page 24

"Responses that stress safety are called coping mechanisms."
>   Kaplan Nursing, Kaplan NCLEX-RN 2014-2015,
>   Strategies, Practice, and Review with Practice Test, page
>   186, Kaplan Inc., 2014

"Caring – As you take the NCLEX-RN, 2014 exam remember that the test is about 'caring' for people, not working with high-tech equipment or analyzing lab results."
>   Kaplan Nursing, Kaplan NCLEX-RN 2014-2015,
>   Strategies, Practices, and Review with Practice Test, page
>   11, Kaplan, Inc., 2014

"The first subcategory for this 'client need' is "Basic Care and Comfort" which accounts for 9 percent of the questions."
>   Kaplan Nursing, Kaplan NCLEX-RN, 2014-2015,
>   Strategies, Practices, and Review with Practice Test, page
>   11, Kaplan Inc., 2014

"Providing basic care and comfort for your clients is one of your most important roles."
>   Kaplan Nursing, Kaplan NCLEX-RN 2014-2015,
>   Strategies, Practice, and Review with Practice Test, page 8,
>   Kaplan Inc., 2014

"Combining medical technology and the 'human touch', health care workers administer care around the clock, responding to the 'needs' of millions of people – from new borns to the critically ill."
>   Health Care, The Big Picture, Chapter 1, Page 1, Video
>   Number 1, JIST Works, America's Career Publisher, The
>   Editors @ JIST, JIST Publishing, 2008

"Anyone considering a career in health care should have a strong desire to help others, genuine concern for the welfare of patients, and clients, and an ability to deal with people of diverse backgrounds in stressful situations."
>   Health-Care Career Vision Book and DVD, page 17, JIST
>   Works, America's Career Publisher, The Editors @ JIST,
>   JIST Publishing, 2008

Here's what it says about Home Health Aides.

"Home Health Aides perform a variety of duties as requested by a client, such as obtaining household supplies or running errands. Accompanying clients to physicians' offices and on other trips from home, providing transportation, assistance, and "companionship". Administer prescribed oral medications under written direction of a physician as directed by home care nurse and aide. Care for children who are disabled or who have sick or disabled parents. Massage patients and apply preparations and treatments such as liniment, alcohol rubs, and heat lamp stimulation."

> Health Care Vision Book and DVD, page 50, JIST Works, America's Career Publisher, The Editors @ JIST, JIST Publishing, 2008

Now that's personal. Talk about me asking nurses to be personal with me. They act like I'm in the wrong for asking for hugs, head rubs, and hand holds. Look what these nurses have to do, the home health aides and nurses.

Along with the long list of duties EMTs and Paramedics are given this is included in the list, "comfort and reassure patients."

> Health Care Vision Book and DVD, page 84, JIST Works, America's Career Publisher, The Editors@JIST, JIST Publishing, 2008

Here is what the Health Care Career Vision Book has to say about Licensed Practical and Licensed Vocational Nurses:

"Care for ill, injured or, 'disabled people', in hospitals, nursing homes, clinics, private homes, group homes, and similar situations."

> Quick Look, page 88, Healthy Care Career Vision Book and DVD, America's Career Publisher, The Editors@JIST, JIST Publishing, 2009

"LPNs provide basic patient care and treatments such as taking temperatures or blood pressures, dressing wounds, treating bed sores, giving enemas, or douches, rubbing with alcohol, 'massaging' or performing Catherizations."

> Health-Care Career Vision Book and DVD, page 88, JIST Works, America's Career Publisher, The Editors@JIST, JIST Publishing, 2008

"Registered Nurses are to 'administer nursing care to ill, injured, convalescent, or 'disabled patients.' They are to 'assess' patient health problems 'and needs', develop and implement nursing care plans and maintain medical records."

> Health-Care Career Vision Book and DVD, page 124, Video 39, JIST Works, America's Career Publisher, The Editors@ JIST, JIST Publishing, 2008

Here are some notes I took on the DVD videos presented on the Health-Care Career Vision Book and DVD videos:

One female nurse rubbed the head of a guy patient while she and the other nurse stood on the sides of his bed. The male patient was wearing a face mask probably for anesthesia to be put to sleep for a procedure.
Another female nurse held a lady patient's hand.

The narrarator made this statement on the DVD.

"For all these jobs you need to be comfortable "touching" the people in your care."

Other things I noticed were as follows:

A female nurse pats a lady patient on the back.

A female nurse holds a guy's hand.

A female nurse put lotion on a patient's foot and rubbed the top of their foot and bottom of their leg.

The narrarator then made this statement on the DVD about Nurse Aides and Orderlies.

"You should have a desire to work with others and have compassion."

On the Video about Licensed Practical Nurses I noted the following:

A female nurse held a male patient's hand.

Another female nurse put her hand on this male patient's shoulder.

Another female nurse held another patient's hand.

The narrarator made the following statement regarding massage therapists on this DVD:

"Being comfortable touching patients is an important necessity."

I believe he also said that many RNS and LPNs give massages as well or at least that they go into massaging during their career.

The narrarator made the following comment about Sonographers:

"Sonographers need to be willing to calm an anxious patient in a comforting way."

The narrarator also made this statement regarding Nuclear Medicine Technologists:

"A friendly reassuring manner is almost more important or better than expertise."

The narrarator made this statement regarding Registered Nurses on the DVD:

"Registered nurses play a crucial role in providing physical and emotional care for the sick, injured, and handicapped."

The narrarator also said, "Registered Nurses have to have a strong desire to help others. You should be compassionate and the well being of patients must be constantly understood and evaluated."

Here are other things I noted about the video on Registered Nurses on the DVD:

A female RN nurse stroked a male patient's face.

The Narrarator said, "RNs must make patients feel at ease before surgery."

He also said, "RNs work in Hospitals, Clinics, and Nursing Homes."

Another female nurse stroked a lady patient's arm before she went for her lab stuff to draw this lady's blood.

I noticed the following on the video about the Physician's Assistants on this DVD:

The narrator said, "P. A. s must be compassionate and caring when working with other people."

About surgeons the narrator said, "Surgeons must have good bedside manner."

I also noticed a surgeon held a patient's hand and put their other hand on the patient's shoulder.

All of this was on the DVD of the Health Care Career Vision Book and DVD. And, by the way, these weren't old, dying people either. They weren't children either. They were my age. I'm 47 years old. They were everyday, middle aged people ages 30s, 40s, and 50s going for procedures and what the DVD showed the nurses do to comfort them in the same manner, by the way, I'm asking them to comfort me. Go see for yourself.

Health-Care Career Vision Book and DVD, DVD Video
Content, JIST Works, America's Career Publisher, The
Editors@JIST, JIST Publishing, 2008

I also found this statement in an AARP magazine. Here's what it
says:

"When you provide another with comfort, when you lend a hand,
or simply be there for someone who needs help, you transform the
health of our country. Big change doesn't require a hero's effort.
Just one small act of kindness can make you a hero to someone
else. How will you participate?"
> Give Health A Hand, Medco Foundation, AARP Magazine,
> March & April 2010, page 67

In Funk & Wagnall's New Illustrated Encyclopedia of Family
Health, 1 A-B, page 60, "a nurse is holding a patient's hand while
giving them anesthesia with a gas mask and holding their stomach
with their other hand."
> Funk & Wagnall's New Illustrated Encyclopedia of Family
> Health, 1, A-B, page 60, The Universal Standard
> Encyclopedia, 1958

"Dr. Diane Meier is quietly leading a revolution to treat patients
(and their families too) as living, breathing, feeling individuals.
And why is that so shocking?"

"When a patient of Diane Mier, MD dies, the family receives a call
or a note. "She was with me when my wife died at home", says
Bert Gold of New York City still missing, Sylvia his wife of 57
years. She took me in the living room and "put her arm around
me" and "started to cry." She "thanked me for letting her take care
of Sylvia. Imagine."
> AARP Magazine, September & October 2007, The
> Comfort Connection by Joan Kenon, page 52, 122, 123

"Meier, 55, of the Mount Sinai School of Medicine in New York School of Medicine in New York City, is one of the leading exponents of a new and growing discipline known as palliative care. Palliative care means soothing the symptoms of a disease, regardless of whether the patient is seeking a cure. It's a concept that's totally transforming the way doctors and hospitals treat seriously ill patients. The ideas of easing pain and improving the quality of a patient's life may seem radical, but classic medical training focuses on attacking the disease. Most doctors simply don't have time to be supersensitive Marcus Welby's checking up on patients to see how they feel. Even if they do have time, they lack the advanced training of palliative care doctors and nurses to ease symptoms such as anxiety, pain, or severe nausea. Most are better equipped to deal with microorganisms than matters of care."
    AARP Magazine, September & October 2007, The
    Comfort Connection by Joan Kenon, page 52, 122, 123

I like Marcus Welby. I think nurses and doctors should be like this again. Besides all this, these nurses may complain they don't have time to comfort their patients but even Gentle Annie and Clara Barton took out the time to comfort their patients in the middle of trying to catch them as they fell off of horses. Soldiers were falling left and right and Clara Barton even cradled a soldier in her arms when he was dying regardless of all the other soldiers around her falling, hoping she could catch them to take care of them. You think you're busy, they were really busy and this never stopped them. They took out time to comfort their patients anyway no matter how busy they were, and that was busy if I ever saw busy.

Try keeping up with that kind of pace with your patients.
That's hard for me to do, and yet I would do this for them too. I just wish you would do this for me.

"When people first hear of palliative care, they often confuse it with Hospice care. Hospice focuses on terminally ill patients, but palliative care teams consist of every one from social worker to physical therapists who can follow patients for days, months, or years."

> AARP Magazine, September & October 2007, The Comfort Connection by Joan Kenon, page 52, 122, 123

"Thanks in large part to the training and outreach programs, Meir runs as the Center for the Advancement of Palliative Care, (CAPC) in New York City, the number of hospitals has nearly doubled, from 632 in 2000 to 1,240 in 2005. Palliative care has the potential to change the way doctors and nurses address pain and emotion, how they help patients and families soothe through their choices as life nears it's end."

> AARP Magazine, September & October 2007, The Comfort Connection by Joan Kenon, page 52, 122, 123

"Bert Gold is 91, takes a lot of medicines, is frail, falls sometimes, lost a big toe, 5 years ago and still deals with pain with an awkward gait. Bert visits Meir in her office today before going back to the foot surgeon and Meir spends 'more than an hour' - yes more than an hour – reviewing his symptoms, his diet, his medications, his mood."

> AARP Magazine, September & October 2007, The Comfort Connection by Joan Kenon, page 52, 122, 123

"Meier believes strongly that palliative care should not be the 'death team', and she sees patients 'early' in the course of the disease."

> AARP Magazine, September & October 2007, The Comfort Connection by Joan Kenon, page 52, 122, 123

"Meir is pushing for more programs and she says 'too many are stuck in a medical no-where land, forced to choose between 'comfort care' and 'emotional support' in a hospice or a chance to keep fighting their illness."
> AARP Magazine, September & October 2007, The Comfort Connection by Joan Kenon, page 52, 122, 123

"Meier says, 'It's not human nature to accept death and agree to give up on life. With palliative care we don't have to."
> AARP Magazine, September & October 2007, The Comfort Connection by Joan Kenon, Health Writer in Washington D.C., page 52, 122, 123

I have seen doctors and nurses comfort their patients on the St. Jude Children's Hospital Commercial several times.

I've even seen a place on the internet I looked up where they had pictures of nurses hugging their patients on a website they had, a whole slew of them.

My mother wanted me to be taken care of after she dies. She wants me to be taken care of and me to be happy and have my needs met.
And, even though my needs seem unusual, my needs are my needs and that is what I need. I'm autistic and I am an Ex-Special Ed student and I have the same childlike needs I had back then. They never went away and they never will and these needs need to be met for the rest of my life. In order for me to be taken care of, I have to be able to get hugs from all my church friends and from all my nurses and doctors and techs when I go to the hospital or doctor's office, and get chipper acting female nurses only who will do this for me, and rub my head to calm me down and hold my hand through all needle sticks every time they're done on me. Meet my list of needs on the list, "all of them" and we are good to go. Please meet my needs.

"The Hebrew Home has put an unusual emphasis on the power of touch and touch therapy. Beverly Herzog has been widowed for 21 years but she still can't get used to this absence. She bought a baby pillow which helps a little but it's not the same. 'I like being touched, being stroked, being held', says Herzog, who lives in the Hebrew Home at Riverdale, a skilled nursing facility in New York. "Anyone who says they don't isn't telling the truth. You feel abandoned if you haven't been touched. We all need somebody." said, Herzog." (Page 38)
> The Power of Touch, pages 37-43, AARP Magazine, December 2015-January 2016

The Hebrew Home has put an unusual emphasis on that idea. The staff here is encouraged to hold resident's hands and offer gentle caresses. Beauticians are trained to massage the feet during pedicures, as well as the scalp and neck during shampoos. And, intimate relationships between residents are not discouraged – a rarity in long term care."
> The Power of Touch, pages 37–43, AARP Magazine, December 2015-January 2016

"Herzog has taken full advantage of this ground breaking policy."
> The Power of Touch, pages 37-43, AARP Magazine, December 2015-January 2016

"When you're younger, it might be easy to take touch for granted. Old people may loose their sense of touch but ironically need to be able to receive touch all the more."
> The Power of Touch, pages 37-43, AARP Magazine, December 2015-January 2016

"Depriving newborns of touch is disaster – growth is slowed, and serious cognitive and behavioral disorders emerge that can persist into adulthood. Touch is crucial for forgoing the first emotional bond with a parent and for creating the unique human experience."
> The Power of Touch, pages 37-43, AARP Magazine, December 2015-January 2016

"Seeing believes", wrote the 18th century English Physician Thomas Fuller, "but Feeling's the truth."
>> The Power of Touch, pages 37-43, AARP Magazine, December 2015-January 2016

"Doctors who touch their patients are not only considered more caring – their patients have better outcomes."
>> The Power of Touch, pages 37-43, AARP Magazine, December 2015-January 2016

"Therapeutic Touch lowers levels of the stress hormone Cortisol and increases the amount of Oxytocin, the so called love hormone, which is credited with mother-and-child bonding, among other things. When we put our hands on each other, we're tapping into deep associations between touch and emotion that are kind let at the dawn of life."
>> The Power of Touch, pages 37-43, AARP Magazine, December 2015-January 2016

This place did more for their residents than I am asking of you. I'm just asking for hugs (putting my right ear on your cheek) from chipper acting, cheery female nurses with motherly personalities when I need to and for you to rub my head to calm me down and hold my hand through needle sticks and I feel like I am being scolded for asking.

"A surrogate- is a substitute figure, especially a person of authority, who replaces a father or mother in one's feelings."
>> Webster's New World Dictionary, 2nd Edition, David B. Garualive, Editor in Chief, William Collins + World Publishing, Co, Inc., 1976

I want all of you, nurses and techs and doctors, and radiologists and anesthesiologists, etc, especially all my nurses and techs to be a surrogate mother to me, especially those working with me. This is what I need.

In response to the quotes on energetics, I believe it is a drawing by the patients you are working with and they are in dire need of your affection or your help to soothe their pain. They are drawing you to them and you are resisting them. I don't believe in any hocus pocus stuff if that's what it is, but I do believe what this woman is saying really happens. I think she just has it mixed up as to what it is and where it is coming from. I think it is a drawing by the patients and by God. They need your help and God would have you to help these people. You are supposed to comfort those in need. I believe they are drawing you to them and God is also drawing you to them and Him. This is what the Bible says about comfort toward others. II Corinthians 1:3,4 says, "Blessed be the God, even the Father of our Lord Jesus Christ, the Father of mercies, and the God of all comfort; who comforteth us in all our tribulation, that we may be able to comfort them which are in any trouble, by the comfort wherewith we ourselves are comforted of God." You see, God expects us to comfort them "which are in any trouble". God is drawing us to him to yield ourselves to help others. My pastor said it himself. I already thought it and tried to decide whether to use this or not, and it came right out of his mouth the very thing I was thinking I want to use to explain to you God's desire for you to meet the needs of others and comfort them in their need, whoever they are, especially your patients. You're a nurse. That's what you're supposed to do. When I see you I get excited and think, "You're going to take care of me! You're going to help me! You're my nurse! You're my friend!" And when you turn the cold shoulder and turn me away when I ask for your comfort or your hugs or long for you to do the same in a non verbal fashion, it tears me apart when you refuse to do this for me. A mother hugs her children and if you are a nurse that acts as a surrogate mother you should be willing to hug your patients and to comfort them through needle sticks. Did not even they who were healed by Jesus cling to him when he healed them? Why do you not let them cling to you when they need you more than anything in their distress? This is what God would have you to do. And, when you comfort them, you need to comfort them in a way that comforts them. If your way does not comfort them it is no comfort at all to them and you need to do what comforts them or they will not be comforted or refreshed.

You can still pat me on the shoulder or rub my shoulder if you wish as some do because I like that too but when another nurse is doing a needle stick on me, I need you to rub my head to calm me down and hold my hand and I always need a hug from both chipper acting, cheery female nurses working with me as well as anyone else I see that I like.

"Nurses have to make people comfortable when they are hurt or afraid."
> Nurses: Community Workers by Cynthia Kingeland, Robert B, Voyed, Compass Point Books, 2003

In the Spanish nurse book Quiero ser Enefermero a nurse rubs the head of a girl that is hooked up to several tubes and EKG leads.
> Quiero Sei Enefermero, Dan Liebman, Firefly Books, 2001

Here are even more examples of movies about nurses in action comforting their patients.

In the movie "Love Finds a Home" Belinda, a doctor takes care of her sister or other doctor friend when she has sharp pains and is pregnant and has a fever. Belinda put her hand on her forehead to see how hot she was. Then she pulled her blanket over her body to cover her. Then, she held her hand. After that she raised her hand up and put it on the lady's face and caressed the side of the lady's face with her hand from the top of her face to the bottom of her face in a stroking motion. Belinda looked at her with deep sadness for her and was filled with compassion. Then she stepped back and let her rest so she could sleep.

I guess some nurses don't think nurses do things like this, but they did here and I've seen several other movies where they did the same kind of thing.

In the movie, "Awakenings", a true story about patients with encephalitis, Dr. Sayre's nurse rubs the old lady patient's head (strokes her head) when she sees how upset she is that it is not still 1922.

Another nurse stroked the top of the head of the red headed lady patient against her hair on the side of her head and then flung her fingers through the strands of her hair at the bottom of her head when she tilted her head backwards to the side in her chair.

Another nurse rubbed a lady patient's upper back in circular motion when they looked at themselves in a mirror and said, "Are you okay?"

If you'll notice, Dr. Sayer him self even gently touched each of his patients as he positioned them as if to show his love for them to make them feel comforted.

On the commercial about St. Jude's Hospital on television they show various ways nurses touch their kid patients to comfort them. I've seen them get close to them several times and either put their arm around them or put their hand on their shoulder. It's hard to remember for sure what all I saw because I haven't seen the commercial in two weeks, so because of that I looked up their commercial videos on the internet and loved what I saw. On the internet video clips of St. Jude's hospital they showed three different nurses hugging their patients. A male nurse was shown hugging their kid patient. Then, a female nurse was shown hugging their kid patient. Then, a toddler ran up to their female nurse and their female nurse hugged them. One female nurse rubbed a kid patient's back.
Another female nurse rubbed a kid patient's hand. One female nurse held a kid patient in their arms.

Another female nurse let a kid patient lay their head on their shoulder. It was wonderful. I thought it was the sweetest thing they did for their kids and it should be that way.

When I looked up nurses comforting patients and clicked on "Images of Nurses Comforting their Patients", I saw a slew of pictures I had to scroll down through showing nurses doing everything for their patients I ever asked you to do. There were about two pages worth of these pictures.

Several nurses held their patients' hands. Several nurses put their hands on their patient's shoulders. One nurse was putting their hand on their patient's back. Another nurse was putting her arm around one of her senior patients. Another nurse put their arm around a kid. The rest of these people were young to middle aged adults. There were a few kids in between, but there must have been at least 15 or 20 pictures of young to middle aged adults in this whole slew of pictures that were getting their hand held, or their shoulder held, and even getting their head rubbed. They even showed one nurse hugging a 37 year old woman. I clicked on this and it went to this story about a New York lady patient getting to reunite with her nurse who took care of her as an infant. The patient's name was Amanda Scrarpauil, and she finally got to meet the nurse that brought her comfort for nearly 40 years. She had a burn she was treated for as a child and she finally got to meet her nurse who took care of her as an infant and be with her again. I have a feeling from the way the rest of the story went she stuck with this nurse from there on out because she loved her so much. This was in the New York Daily Times on the computer.

Bertha just recently got a miniature magazine similar to a Reader's Digest book called "Prayer Point - Summer 2016." On the cover of this little miniature magazine you will see a nurse putting her hand on the head of a female patient and leaning her face down toward her looking at her with concern while she is laying in a bed hooked up to an IV. This book has the title at the bottom "Life Saving Compassion."

You can't tell me nurses don't rub their patients heads to calm them down, especially after I already saw the exact same thing on the Health Care Career DVD from 2008 of them doing this for patients "my age" (not dying ones, but sick ones). They showed them rub their heads too, several times. The same thing was shown on the Facing Death DVD of the patients that really were dying, but they don't have to be dying for them to do this, they do it anyway for all ages, when they do they're job right and don't complain it's not in their job description to do so.

When I looked up "Nurses Hugging Patients, or Nurses Giving Patients Hugs" on the Internet and clicked on Images of Nurses Hugging Patients, there were several of them, probably two pages worth of pictures of nurses hugging their patients.

When I looked up videos on nursing it was harder to find what I was looking for because they were mainly showing the technical stuff for educational purposes to show nurse students how to take a blood test or take records for example, but there was one I found from VC San Diego Medical Center where two chipper acting female nurses were taking care of a lady while another nurse sat at her bedside and held her hand. Then, when the two chipper acting nurses began working with the lady patient one of these two chipper acting female nurses put their hands on the patient's shoulder when she asked a question. Then she put her hand on her arm to tell her something. When she wanted to check her response ability, she told this lady, "Squeeze my hand when I say "A". She began Saying, "A. S. A. S. A. A." every time she said "A" the lady patient squeezed her hand. This nurse was very sweet and had the type of personality I like in a nurse. She was very chipper and sweet and caring. I thought it was great.

On one of these videos they had a box of words to the side that said, "To Care", "To Advocate", "To Inspire", "To Be a Nurse", "Nursing."

When I looked up a video on needle phobics, one nurse was stating, "You need to be more than careful when dealing with a needle phobic patient. They need a lot of attention."
She went on to say, "When they come for me to take blood, I'm going to lay them down. I'm not going to have them sit in my chair."

I've always requested the nurses lay me down to draw blood because that works better for me. Some lab techs or nurses will do this for me, but there have been some who didn't understand and wanted to use their chair anyway because they cared more about whether it suited them or the doctor more to do it in the chair than they did about whether it suited me.

It works better to lay me down on a bed to do it. And, when you do, one chipper acting female nurse needs to stand on the left side of the bed to rub my head to calm me down and hold my hand while another chipper acting female nurse does the Blood test, IV, or shot in the right arm because it hurts worse to do it in the left. Also, when it comes to shots, I don't mean to embarrass anybody, but it hurts less to have those in the hip so anytime you can do those in the hip please do. I haven't had a shot in the arm for close to 25 years and I have a feeling I'd jump and freak out for sure if you attempted to give me a shot there again. And, I know you probably think I'm a cry baby for this, because you're thinking, "It's only a shot", but I want a chipper acting female nurse to stand to the side of me to rub my head to calm me down while the other chipper acting female nurse does the shot too. And, all you other doctor offices and hospital staff out there, I need you to do this for me too. I need you to do this for the shot, and the blood test, and the IV, and anything else sharp, even biopsies, or anything invasive, please. It's very important you do this for me. And, my new doctor, technically a nurse practitioner, wanted to do one of those allergy tests on me when she gets the equipment to do it with and poke me with one of those multipronged metal things. I hope she doesn't mind, but I need the chipper acting girl that works for her to rub my head to calm me down and hold my hand when she does it, because it is also scary to me. I'm hoping she doesn't think, "It's not even a needle. It's just a prong device." But it has several point sharp ends on it and it's scary to even think about how much that might hurt, because I have oversensitivity to pain and I'm scared that's really going to hurt. I'm almost more afraid of it than I am the needle.

I also saw a nurse give a patient a hug on one of my video tapes, and in one place saw a picture of a nurse hugging a patient. Here is another example of what I have seen in one of my movies that were just lying around the house.

In the Feature Films for Families movie, "Alan and Naomi" about the shy girl that got continually panicked in public especially in crowds, after a nurse took Naomi to the Mental Hospital and they showed Naomi sitting on a bench, they also showed one of the nurses hug one of their patients in the field and afterwards they leaned the patient's head on their shoulder and gently put their hand against their head in the front yard of the mental health hospital.

My definition of comfort has always been "to cheer up and show affection to" by talking with an uplifting spirit to your patients and give them hugs, and rub their head to calm them down through needle sticks, and hold their hand, and pat them on the shoulder and rub their shoulder, etc. I've seen this my whole life as the definition of comfort from everyone including parents, friends, teachers, nurses, doctors, techs, church friends, and other acquaintances.

My whole life I've see it this way, and now some of these nurses seem to want to redefine comfort as if it is something else. Comfort to me is what it has always been, a warm hug, a tender touch, or a rub on the head or shoulder.
None of this other stuff they come up with these days is comfort. It's just a lame excuse to get out of showing comfort so they don't have to get too personal with you when in reality that's what nursing is all about, mothering your patients helping heal their wounds and comforting them in their sorrow and pain.

Even if they are not in sorrow or pain, they will be if you don't comfort them because they will feel like you don't care and they're just a number to you, and they are starved for affection because you didn't give it to them and their heart is broken. Is that really what you want?

Refusing to comfort your patients is wrong, and any patient that comes to you should be able to be comforted by you if they ask you to comfort them whether you feel like they need it or not.

They just need to feel loved and cared for and you are supposed to treat your patients as a mother treats their own children. Not doing so just causes chaos and fear and broken heartedness and even if you stood a chance of saving your patient you may have just lost them because of what you just did. You refused them of the very thing they needed. The comfort they needed you to give them as you would give to your own child. Please comfort your patients, especially me. It especially causes chaos when a patient has a sensory issue in their right ear like me that can only be relieved by putting it on the cheek of the people that I like, including nurses. The disabled need it worse than ever. They need their needs met even worse than normal every day people do and when you keep that from them it traumatizes them and causes them to lose their will to live. They feel like me, like why bother getting well if my nurses are going to treat me like a stranger they just want to fix up and get rid of. They're just there for the paycheck and they don't care anything about me. Why doesn't anybody care? Please remember to show compassion in your care and comfort your patients the way they need comforted. Thank you.

Just as Solomon in the Bible told God that he wanted wisdom instead of riches, I wish to have affection instead of riches including my hugs from my church friends and my doctors and nurses and techs at all my doctor's offices and every department in the hospital that I see, especially those taking care of me.

I still want to have a feasible income, but I would rather receive all the affection I need, especially the hugs I need from everyone everywhere I go, especially at church and at the doctor's offices and hospitals I go to than to have riches galore. I only ask I get my need for hugs and affection met and can live feasibly enough financially to get by. In the medical setting this means I get my hugs I need from all my nurses and doctors and techs, and that the chipper acting female nurses I get rub my head to calm me down and hold my hand through needle sticks. You give me that, and we've got it made.

Male nurses, doctors, and techs tortured me as a child, and serious trended female nurses tortured me in both childhood and adulthood.

Only the chipper ones ever showed me the compassion and comfort I needed and they are the ones I need because they have the chipperness I need to cheer me up and the compassion to comfort me the way I ask them to comfort me with motherly love.

Some nurses may say, "It's not going to kill you if we don't do this for you." Bertha was starved when she was a kid and she didn't die either, but she got food eventually. Had Bertha never got any food ever again, eventually, it would have caught up with her and she would have died from starvation had she not eventually got something to eat after being starved. Just as that is true for her, you may refuse to hug me once and it may not kill me, but refuse me consistently one too many times and it could cause me to die of a broken heart. It is that traumatic for me. The last time Bertha was an inpatient in a hospital the nurses that knew me in that department were gone. They had all quit their jobs. Instead, all these stoic acting nurses were working in there that did not understand. All of them refused to hug me. Then, two more nurses refused to hug me in the kitchen. I was crying and walking slowly and started having tremors and could barely hold on to my food. The cashier finally said, "Do you need a tray?" I finally said, "Yeah." and slowly walked out of there. She didn't know the reason I was having tremors was because I was that upset I couldn't get any hugs and it spooked me to be stuck in a place for 24 hours with no hugs with Bertha in the bed and I couldn't get out of there. I was trapped. The nurse in charge of these other nurses noticed something was wrong and kept asking me if I was okay. She acted like she knew something wasn't right, because I wasn't acting my normal self. I barely ate what I got, even though I got something to eat that I liked because it upset me so bad that I could not get hugs and could not wait to get out of there but felt trapped. This nurse noticed how slowly I barely ate what I had even though it was something I liked to eat and knew something had to be wrong. She actually begged me to eat and said, "Please, you need to eat something. I'm really worried."

This is how badly it upsets me to not have hugs and if too many people refuse me hugs for too long I go into crying fits and start having panic attacks and lose my will to live.

Have you ever seen "Cipher in the Snow"? He felt like he wasn't good enough for anybody and nobody wanted him. He felt like he had no friends. One day, he asked the bus driver, "Excuse me can I get off the bus for a minute. I need a break." The bus driver stopped the bus in the middle of nowhere and said, "Sure."
The kid walked off the bus and stepped down to the ground into the snow and passed out on the spot and died of a broken heart. That's what you do to me when you do this to me.

I was getting to the point where I was so frustrated with the last few doctors and nurses I had to deal with not being willing to meet my needs that I was never going to go to the doctor again. That was even after I finally got all new specialist's offices that were willing to meet my needs but the last family doctor I went to was not. They could have taken care of most things, but there was some things left over I still had to go to a family doctor for such as my problem with anemia and my B12 deficiency and a few other miscellaneous problems I have you don't normally go to a specialist for.

I finally found a family doctor after this one, that is actually a nurse practitioner who was very nice to me and very understanding to me and promised to meet all my needs in her office including the hugs I am asking for and be willing to have her assistant rub my head to calm me down and hold my hand through a needle stick. She's even going to try to set me up with one last specialist I don't have yet that I need that she thinks will understand me and she says their nurse is really nice and very understanding and she thinks I would really like this lady. And, if she can't get me in there, she has other places she's going to try until she finds one that will take me and meet all my needs on my list of needs. I'm hoping I finally have all doctors and nurses and a hospital that will meet my needs and give me the hugs I need and be willing to rub my head to calm me down and hold my hand through an IV stick, blood test, shot, or biopsy, or anything else sharp or invasive.

If I do, I don't have anything to worry about. I was starting to get worried, but now I think we've got it fixed. I hope I'm right. Please see to it that you meet my needs. Thanks. I need all my doctors and nurses at my doctor's offices and the nurses and techs and doctors and radiologists and anesthesiologists at the hospital to meet my entire list of needs. This is very important to me and not doing so traumatizes me.

To Nurse means to nurture and any nurse that is not willing to comfort their patients like they would their child or baby should not be a nurse and find a different profession to work in.

"As nurses deal with health and illness in their practice they grow in the ability to care. Nursing behaviors related to caring include providing presence, a "caring touch", and "listening". Nurses who demonstrate caring use a caring approach in each encounter with clients."
> Fundamentals of Nursing, 7th Edition, page 100, Potter and Perry, Mosby Elsevier, 2009

"Providing presence is a person to person encounter conveying a closeness and a sense of caring. Fredrickson (1999) explains that presence involves "being there" and "being with". Being there is not only a physical presence, but also includes communication and understanding."
> Fundamentals of Nursing, 7th Edition, page 100, Potter and Perry, Mosby Elsevier, 2009

"The interpersonal relationship of "being there" seems to depend on the clients (Cohen and others, 1994)."
> Fundamentals of Nursing, 7th Edition, page 100, Potter and Perry, Mosby Elsevier, 2009

"This type of presence is something the nurse offers to the client with the purpose of achieving some goal, such as support, "comfort", or encouragement to diminish the intensity of unwanted feelings, or for reassurance (Fareed, 1996; Pedersen, 1993)"
> Fundamentals of Nursing, 7th Edition, pages 100,101, Potter and Perry, Mosby Elsevier, 2009

"Being with" is also interpersonal. The nurse gives himself, or herself which means being available and at a client's disposal (Pedersen 1993). If clients accept the nurse, the will invite him or her to see, share and "touch" their vulnerability and suffering."

> Fundamentals of Nursing, 7th Edition, page 101, Potter and Perry, Mosby Elsevier, 2009

"It is especially important to establish presence when clients are experiencing stressful events or situations."

> Fundamentals of Nursing, 7th Edition, page 101, Potter and Perry, Mosby Elsevier, 2009

"The nurse's presence helps to calm anxiety and fear related to stressful situations. Giving reassurance and thorough explanations about a procedure, "remaining at the client's side", and "coaching the client through the experience" all convey a presence that is invaluable to the client's well being."

> Fundamentals of Nursing, 7th Edition, page 101, Potter and Perry, Mosby Elsevier, 2009

"Clients face situations that are embarrassing, frightening, and painful. Whatever the feeling or symptom, clients look to nurses to "provide comfort". The "use of touch" is one "comforting approach" where the nurse "reaches out to clients to communicate concern and support."

> Fundamentals of Nursing, 7th Edition, page 101, Potter and Perry, Mosby Elsevier, 2009

"Touch is relational and leads to a connection between nurse and client. Touch involves contact and noncontact touch (Frederickson, 1999). Contact touch involves obvious skin-to-skin contact, whereas noncontact touch refers to eye contact. It is difficult to separate the two. Both in turn are described within three categories: task-oriented touch, caring touch, and protective touch (Fredrickson 1999)."

> Fundamentals of Nursing, 7th Edition, page 101, Potter and Perry, Mosby Elsevier, 2009

"Nurses use task-oriented touch when performing a task or procedure. The skillful and gentle performance of a nursing procedure conveys security and a sense of competence. An expert nurse learns that any procedure is more effective when administered carefully and in consideration of any client concern. For example, if a client is anxious about having a procedure, such as the insertion of a nasogastric tube, the nurse offers "comfort" through a full explanation of the procedure and what the client will feel."

> Fundamentals of Nursing, 7th Edition, page 101, Potter and Perry, Mosby Elsevier, 2009

"The nurse then expresses that the procedure will be performed safely, skillfully, and successfully. This is done in the way that supplies are prepared, the client is positioned, and the nasogastric tube is gently manipulated and inserted. Throughout a procedure the nurse talks quietly with the client to provide assurance and support."

> Fundamentals of Nursing, 7th Edition, page 101, Potter and Perry, Mosby Elsevier, 2009

"Caring touch is a form of nonverbal communication, which successfully influences a client's comfort and security, enhances self-esteem, and improves reality orientation (Boyek and Watson, 1994). You express this in the way you "hold a client's hand", "give a back massage", "gently position a client", "or "participate in a conversation."

> Fundamentals of Nursing, 7th Edition, page 101, Potter and Perry, Mosby Elsevier, 2009

"When using a "caring touch", the nurse is making a connection with the client and showing acceptance of the individual (Tommansini, 1990)."

> Fundamentals of Nursing, 7th Edition, page 101, Potter and Perry, Mosby Elsevier, 2009

"Protective touch is a form of touch used to protect the nurse and/or client (Fredriksson, 1999). The client views it either positively or negatively. The most obvious form of protective touch is preventing an accident, for example, holding and bracing the client to avoid a fall. Protective touch is also a kind of touch that protects the nurse emotionally."

>Fundamentals of Nursing, 7th Edition, page 101, Potter and Perry, Mosby Elsevier, 2009

"The client generally permits task-oriented touch, because most individuals give nurses and physicians a license to enter their personal space to provide care. Know and understand if clients are accepting of touch and how they interpret the nurse's intentions."

>Fundamentals of Nursing, 7th Edition, page 101, Potter and Perry, Mosby Elsevier, 2009

That says the "nurse's intentions, not the patients. So, in other words, it's the other way around from what nurses have been telling me the past couple of years. This book is not asking me to okay touch with you, it is asking you to okay touch with me, and it says you are supposed to touch me if I want you to touch me and say I need you to touch me.

"Caring involves an interpersonal interaction that is much more that two persons simply talking back and forth. In a caring relationship the nurse establishes trust, opens lines of communication and listens to what the client has to say. Listening is key because it conveys the nurse's full attention and interest."

>Fundamentals of Nursing, 7th Edition, page 101, Potter and Perry, Mosby Elsevier, 2009

"Listening includes "taking in" what a client says, as well as interpretation and understanding of what the client is saying and giving back that understanding to the person talking (Kemper, 1992)."

>Fundamentals of Nursing, 7th Edition, page 101, Potter and Perry, Mosby Elsevier, 2009

"Listening to the meaning of what a client says helps create a mutual relationship. True listening leads to truly knowing and responding to what really matters to the client and family (Boykin and others, 2003)."

> Fundamentals of Nursing, 7th Edition, page 101, Potter and Perry, Mosby Elsevier, 2009

"Caring is a moral imperative. Through caring for other human beings, ultimately human dignity is protected, enhanced, and preserved. Watson (1988) suggests that caring, as a moral ideal, provides the stance from which one intervenes as a nurse."

> Fundamentals of Nursing, 7th Edition, page 100, Potter and Perry, Mosby Elsevier, 2009

"Showing the family care and concern for the client creates an openness that then enables a relationship to form with the family. Caring for the family takes into consideration the context of the client's illness and the stress it imposes on all members."

> Fundamentals of Nursing, 7th Edition, page 103 Pottery and Perry, Mosby Elsevier, 2009

"An ethics of care is concerned with relationships between people and with a nurse's character and attitude toward others. Nurses who function from an ethic of care are sensitive to unequal relationships that lead to an abuse of one person's power over another – intentional or otherwise."

> Fundamentals of Nursing, 7th Edition, page 100, Potter and Perry, Mosby Elsevier, 2009

In health care settings clients and families are often on unequal footing with professionals because of the client's illness, lack of information, regression caused by pain, and unfamiliar circumstances."

> Fundamentals of Nursing, 7th Edition, page 100, Potter and Perry, Mosby Elsevier, 2009

I've been in hospitals before where the nurses at that hospital acted like they thought they somehow dominated over me because they were a nurse and I had to do everything they said and couldn't do a thing about it if they decided they wanted to do something painful to me and not be nice about it and show me no mercy in my pain. One time, after having to go to several steps just to get me sat up in a hospital bed, and put me in excruciating pain in the process, and then having even more trouble getting me sat up, much less walked to a chair, two nurses complained about having to give me a bath and were mean about getting me out of bed and handled me very roughly. They both yelled out, "You could have done this yourself if you wanted to!" One of them was much more hateful than the other one was. The meanest nurse asked the other one the question, "Why is it hurting him so much?" when they tried to get me sat up in the bed. The other nurse said, "I don't know." I was temporarily in an invalid state because I just had prostate surgery and had a catheter in me, and I was already in excruciating pain from having it in me, but even worse, the least little pull you did to it, it would put me in agonizing, unbearable excruciating pain unlike anything you ever saw. Now, for my next point, after they bathed me, they left me sitting in the chair. Before the meanest nurse of the two left the room left she noticed how horrible a time I was having getting around and figured out I was not faking it. This lady suddenly got mad and ugly when she was done with me and said, "You'd better hope your doing better than this in three days or you'll never get out of here, so you better hope your doing better in three days or your not going anywhere!" Then she proceeded to say, "I'm going to come back in here later, and I'm going to drag you out of that bed and I'm going to walk you down that hall, so you'd better be ready!" I panicked and begged and pleaded with her and said, "Please. Don't make me do it again. It's too hard for me to handle. I can't handle doing this again. Can you just walk me down the hall now so we can have this over with?" The lady said, "Hold on. Let me go down here and find out if I can walk you now or not and I'll be back in 20 minutes." The lady never returned, and I was left in the chair alone. I think someone finally helped me get back in my patient bed way later.

Then while I was back in the bed I called the Charge nurse and complained about this lady and said, "Your nurse said she was going to come in here and drag me out of the bed and walk me down the hall. Please, don't make me do it. I can't handle doing it again." The Charge nurse then said, "Oh, you probably could, but it would be very painful." (Sarcastically). I felt like I was this nurse's prisoner and that she thought I was her prisoner and I felt like the Charge nurse thought I was too. Later all three of them readjusted my catheter several times over putting me in excruciating pain acting like they got a thrill out of it and did this for several minutes against my will. The Charge nurse at that hospital even started making sarcastic comments to me like, "You know, if you're in here for more than three days we're going to have to reinsert that IV" and "You know, if you're in here for more than three days, we're going to have to reinsert that catheter." Acting like she was about to cackle when she said it.
I said, "No, no! Please! Don't make me do it! Don't let them make me redo the catheter awake! Make sure they send me to PreOp to put me back to sleep first before they reinsert it!" The Charge nurse sarcastically said, "It depends. They may do want you want them to, but they may not either. If they don't you'll just have to let them do it and you'll have to do it for them." On the day I was to leave, after I got disconnected from all my stuff I offered to take my own bath so these other nurses wouldn't have to bathe me. I wanted to make everybody happy and she said, "Not without a nurse's assistance you're not!" I got tired of waiting for them to let me bathe and after a couple of hours I walked down to the nurses station and she saw me in my hospital gown and looked at me like she was trying to make me self-conscious that I was only wearing a hospital gown and started laughing at me and then all the other nurses at the station she was at starting laughing at me with her. She even made it as impossible as she possibly could for me to get discharged from the hospital on my last day there, and made fun of me when I went to talk to her, and got everyone else to laugh at me with her. And they wound up doing it for me anyway. I couldn't win either way. If they were going to make me let them help me to start with, then what were they complaining about the first time.

When I tried to sign papers after the doctor was already supposed to have discharged me, one nurse said, "What do you want?" I said, "I was told I could go home as soon as I signed the discharge papers." Then another nurse said, "Where do you think you're going?" I said, "I just want to go home. The doctor said I could go home now." The nurse said, "It will be a while! Go back to your room!" rudely. This is an example of how they can exceed their power and take control over their patients by abusing their power of authority as a nurse. This is one of the biggest reasons I don't like serious trended female nurses. They always do this to me. They act like they think I'm their property and they can kick me around all they want and I can't do anything about it, but give me over to a chipper acting cheery female nurse who understands and things work out a whole lot differently than what you've seen happen here. This was terrible, and I never want a male nurse or serious trended female nurse again.

They don't care about my oversensitivy to pain either and if I don't already have an IV or catheter in from where someone nicer already inserted it and they get a hold of me, they will manhandle me to get it done and be mean about it and gripe and complain about my screaming and squeamishness and give me all kinds of havoc and not care that they are hurting me. They're not nice like the chipper nurses are. At least the chipper acting ones try to sweet talk me into letting them stick me or insert things in me and are nice about it and try to comfort me through it, but these serious trended types are terrors when it comes to needle sticks and other invasive procedures. And, when I was a kid if I was afraid of them and I tried to refuse to cooperate with them they forced me to cooperate with them no matter what it meant. And these people in this story were nurses I ran into in my adulthood only a little over a decade ago, so since they were already rough with what they did do, I think if the rest had not been done by someone else they would have been just as mean and meaner if they would have been the ones to prep me. I think it was quite obvious they would have been because of how big a kick out of it this charge nurse got out of the possibility she might be able to put me in pain by reinserting stuff and this other lady that worked with me was already rough with me as it was, let her at something like this and I guarantee you disaster would have happened.

This happens almost every time I get either one of them, and neither one of them have the motherly compassion of a chipper acting cheerful motherly female nurse to show me the affection I need and the comfort and consolation I need to get through procedures and inpatient stays. They are always the best and they are the ones that make me happy, and they are the one's I am comfortable with.

"An ethic of care places the "nurse" as the "patient's advocate", solving ethical dilemmas by attending to relationships and by giving priority to each client's unique personhood."
> Fundamentals of Nursing, 7th Edition, page 100, Potter and Perry, Mosby Elsevier, 2009

"When an individual becomes ill, he or she usually has a story to tell about the meaning of their illness. Any critical or chronic illness affects all of a client's life choices and decisions, sometimes affecting the individual's identity. Being able to tell that story helps the client break the distress of illness."
> Fundamentals of Nursing, 7th Edition, page 102, Potter and Perry, Mosby Elsevier, 2009

"The experienced nurse knows additional facts about his or her clients such as their experiences, behaviors, feelings, and perceptions (Radwin, 1995). When you make clinical decisions accurately in the context of knowing a client well, improved client outcomes will result. Swanson (1999b) notes that when nurses base care on knowing the client, the clients perceive care as personalized, comforting, supportive, and healing."
> Fundamentals of Nursing, 7th Edition, page 102, Potter and Perry, Mosby Elsevier, 2009

"To know a client is to enter into a caring, social process that results in a "bonding" whereby the client comes to feel known by the nurse (Lamb and Stempel, 1994)."
> Fundamentals of Nursing, 7th Edition, page 102, Potter and Perry, Mosby Elsevier, 2009

"The bonding then sets the stage for the relationship to evolve into "working" and "changing" phases so that you help the client become involved in his or her care and accept help when needed (Bulfin, 2005)."

> Fundamentals of Nursing, 7th Edition, page 102, Potter and Perry, Mosby Elsevier, 2009

I like the way the two chipper acting female nurses in Figure 4-3, page 54, Basic Nursing: A Psychophysiologic Approach, Sorenson & Luckman, 1979 are taking care of an infant by comforting them and playing with them and smiling at them sweetly. This is what I would like. I know I'm not an infant, but I am autistic and have the mental capacity of a child in the area of social and emotional issues and this is what I need. I may be intellectually smart, but I am still sociably and emotionally like a 5-year-old with the communication skills of an 8 to 10 year old and I have a record from a lady that tested me for Autism during adulthood to prove it. I'm like below average to average in the area of book smarts and borderline in the areas of spatial perception, socialization, emotional feelings, and areas of functional performance. And, I should be able to get this kind of special attention and have my special needs met from all chipper acting female nurses only and no one else the way I need them met. It actually traumatizes me not to meet my needs and what I ask for is what works for me and what works the best and is the only thing that works. Nothing else outside of what I ask helps. I ask for what I need and that is what I need and those needs need to be met.

"Caring is a motivating force for people to become nurses, and it becomes the source of satisfaction when nurses know they have made a difference in their clients' lives."

> Fundamentals of Nursing, 7th Edition, page 102, Potter and Perry, Mosby Elsevier, 2009

"The study of clients'' perceptions is important because health care is placing greater emphasis on client satisfaction. When clients sense that health care providers are sensitive, sympathetic, compassionate, and interested in them as people, they usually become active partners in the plan of care (Atttree, 2001)."

> Fundamentals of Nursing, 7th Edition, pages 99, 100, Perry and Potter, Mosby Elsevier, 2009

"In health care settings, meaningful touch is limited, environments lack sensory stimulatory properties, meals are dull and bland, and bath times are unpleasant and distressing experiences (MacDonald, 2002).

> Fundamentals of Nursing, 7th Edition, page 100, Perry and Potter, Mosby Elsevier, 2009

"When a person experiences an inadequate quality or quantity of stimulation, such as monotonous or meaningless stimuli, sensory depravation occurs."

> Fundamentals of Nursing, 7th Edition, page 100, Perry and Potter, Mosby Elsevier, 2009

With me I have overstimulation in my right ear because of some kind of weird sensory stimulus in my ear I've had since birth that can only be relieved by putting it on the cheek of the person I like. Because of this overstimulation in my right ear that can only be offset from being able to press it on the cheek of the person I like, when a person refuses to give me a hug it throws me into overstimulation of the ear from not getting to hug somebody I like and throws me into sensory depravation by not getting the need met I need met by getting to put my right ear on someone's cheek when this happens.

In the hospital or doctor's office setting that would be the nurse I am asking to do this for me and when they refuse I am depraved of touch in the way I need touched most of all by not being able to give them a hug by putting my right ear on their cheek which soothes the sensation I have in my ear and tames it down and relieves it.

It's like taking Pepto Bismol to soothe a person's stomach when it is inflamed which tames it down, calms it, soothes it, and relieves it. I also have oversensitivity to pain and need comforted through needle sticks. The chipper acting cheery female nurse needs to rub my head to calm me down and hold my hand while the other chipper acting cheery female nurse does the IV, Blood Test, Shot, Biopsy, Incision, or use of any other sharp object is used on me. This is what helps me and this is what I need.

"Care of clients at risk for sensory deprivation includes introducing meaningful and pleasant stimuli for all senses".
> Fundamentals of Nursing, 7th Edition, page 1362, Potter and Perry, Mosby Elsevier, 2009

"When conducting an assessment, review the client's expectations. Many clients have a definite plan as to how they want their care delivered. Some clients expect caregivers to recognize and appropriately manage and adjust their environment to meet their sensory needs. This includes assisting the individual client in learning and adapting to a changed lifestyle based on the specific sensory impairment."
> Fundamentals of Nursing, 7th Edition, page 1362, Potter and Perry, Mosby Elsevier, 2009

"Determine from clients exactly what they expect to achieve and what interventions have been helpful in the past in the management of any limitation. Always remember that clients with sensory alterations have strengthened their other senses and expect caregivers to anticipate their needs (e.g. for safety and security)."
> Fundamentals of Nursing, 7th Edition, page 1362, Potter and Perry, Mosby Elsevier, 2009

I can't handle not being able to hug people I like, especially when I am in a hospital based situation where something medical is going on with either me or Bertha, especially if I'm the one going through the experience. I need the comfort of others to feel at ease when I go for stuff like this instead of being treated like I'm some stranger over here that you really don't want to get too close to.

I can't handle you just wanting to shun away or you try to greet me like I'm someone at some firm somewhere.

My need to hug is actually a sensory issue I have that has to be met in order for me to be able to function like everyone else. I have to be able to put my right ear on the cheek of the person I like for comfort to offset the sensation I get in my ear to make it go away. This soothes my ear, and putting it on someone's cheek feels like putting it on a soft pillow. The softness of the person's cheek helps to soothe my ear to make the uncomfortable sensation go away in my ear and makes me feel better. I also feel like the people who do this for me by letting me do this care about me because I feel like they care how I feel, and I feel like they are my friends, even if they are an acquaintance. I really appreciate it when they do this for me. I really need this from people I like something tremendous and always have. I have always required a lot of affection my whole life. It's not my fault I make people feel like I'm a nuisance to them. And, I know some of you may say, "If it feels like a pillow, why don't you just lay on a pillow?" but like the lady in the article I wrote about that was in the AARP article about touch, a pillow is still not a good substitute even though it does help some, because there is something about the sensation in my ear that can only be relieved by putting it on the cheek of the person's face. Regardless of the fact, it feels similar to a pillow, there's still something extra special about it that does a much better job of soothing my ear and making the sensation go away.

You know how autistic people have some kind of weird thing about "textures", something about the texture of the cheek, has a certain softness about it you cannot find anywhere else that if I want the sensation in my ear to go away, I have to be able to touch with my ear because it is the only way to make it go away, because even though a pillow may or may not help someone, the sensation will never really go away unless I place my right ear on someone's cheek. It's really weird, but it's true. Some of you have seen how desperate I am to receive a hug from you or give you a hug when I'm laying down in a patient bed and I'm laying on a pillow then. When I get the sensation to hug somebody, the pillow does not do any good, and the only way I can relieve the uncomfortable sensation is to be able to place it on the cheek of the person I like, especially the nurse that's working with me.

120

This is also true with any other nurses I see I like whether they are working with me or not. Not being able to do so sends me into chaos and I constantly long for and reach for you to give me a hug because I need one. I need to be able to hug who I like whether I'm scared or not, but when I am scared I need to be able to hug you worse than ever or I will not feel at ease. I will be stressed beyond anything you've ever seen and fall into a deep depression because it is that detrimental I get this need met by the people I like, including nurses and techs and doctors and radiologists and anesthesiologists, anyone in the medical field and my friends. I will always need this. Not being able to do so for an extended period of time causes me to lose my will to live. I think if you knew it was that serious and that important I get to hug you, you would probably rather cave in and give me a hug than to take a chance on sending me into so deep a depression you almost lose me. Plus, I would be very upset if you didn't. Chances are, I probably wouldn't stick around and you'd be without a patient if you did refuse me a hug. I really need this. Please make sure to do this for me. Autistic people have sensory things that have to be met a certain way in order to offset the uncomfortable sensation they are having. It's like pouring water on someone's burning tongue, or putting anti-itch cream on someone's arm that itches, or putting someone's hands under water in the sink after they've burned themselves on a stove, or someone cooling their face off in front of a window air conditioner after they've been out in the extreme heat for a long time. It's also like someone brushing their teeth to get the yuck or stink or sleep taste out of their mouth, or, better yet, someone taking Pepto Bismol or Mylanta to soothe the stomach after experiencing indigestion, inflammation, or ulcer pain. Giving someone a hug and placing my right ear on their cheek is like taking the Pepto Bismol to soothe the stomach when it's irritated. The Pepto Bismol soothes the stomach and tames it down and that's what getting to hug somebody does for me. If someone asked you, "Could I have a piece of chocolate cake?" would you say, "Here, have a cracker." when it is in your means to be able to give them a piece of chocolate cake. I didn't think so.

When people try to force me to shake their hand or bump arms instead of hugging me because it's the way they want to do it because the hugging thing doesn't seem normal to them, they don't realize that when they do this to me, that it would be like you wanting to brush your teeth to get the yuck out of your mouth and then someone say to you "I'll give you a mint." And you say, "But I want toothpaste. I know a mint might put a nice flavor in your mouth but that still doesn't get rid of the stink in my mouth." And, they say to you, "I'm sorry. You can't have toothpaste and a toothbrush to brush your teeth with. I'm only giving you a mint." If they did this, they would think they were justifying themselves for making you do what they want you to do instead of meeting your actual need, because the mint, in their mind is supposed to freshen your breath. But, that mint is not going to be able to get that stuff off your teeth to make you able to feel clean and refreshed and be totally rid of the yuck taste feeling in your mouth until you get your toothpaste and brush your teeth with a toothbrush and toothpaste. Without the toothpaste, your need to get that gunk off your teeth will never be met, because you won't be able to get it off without it. You may be able to temporarily keep your mouth from stinking someone else out, but you will never get that gunk off your teeth until someone gives you the toothpaste you ask for to get it off of there.

So, when someone refuses to give me a hug and asks me to shake their hand instead, it's like making you settle for a mint instead of giving you the toothpaste you asked them for. You may have asked them for the toothpaste because it is what you wanted, and they may see it as a want, but in reality what you asked for is really a need. You may want it, and it is true that you were asking for something you wanted, but what you wanted was also what you needed, and that was the toothpaste you asked for that was going to get that gunk off of your teeth. Without getting the toothpaste, the mint is of no use, because the mint is only candy, not a gunk remover, and without the toothpaste the gunk will never come off your teeth no matter how many mints you eat. This is what people do when they refuse me a hug, but it is even worse than this; it is so horrible that it is like refusing to give someone a teaspoon of Pepto Bismol to soothe their stomach pain.

Without it their stomach will ever be inflamed and in pain and agony. When they receive it they get relief and it tames their stomach down and makes it calm and at ease. When someone gives me a hug, it calms down the sensory output that causes me to need a hug and tames it down in such a way that it is like soothing a person's stomach with Pepto Bismol. If this confuses you as to what it feels like, a hug doesn't feel like a bottle of medicine if you're taking it literally. A hug just has a medicinal like affect on me when I am able to hug someone. When I press my right ear on your cheek it feels similar to what it feels like to lay your head on a feather pillow, especially the part of your face I put my right ear on. It is very soothing and very calming and helps me to stabilize myself. I was born like this. It has never been any other way. I have been like this and had this kind of sensory issue all 47 years of my life that I've been alive. There is nothing new about it. It has always been this way and always will be this way. I have always needed hugs this way and will always need hugs this way, and unfortunately for some people who get tired of it, I actually need several hugs a day from every person I meet that I like. It is that serious a thing. I actually have to have this or it will send me into a physically chaotic state of some kind. I'm not sure how to describe it, but like I said, it's like putting someone's hand under cool water after they accidentally burn it on the stove; you have to put it under cool water several times throughout the day, especially the first few minutes or few hours after the burn accident occurs. You have to do this, no matter who you are, or you will be in serious trouble from your burn and it will get detrimentally worse if you don't. You have to cool it under water several times or you will be in trouble. You have no choice. You have to do this because it is detrimental you have this done. Not cooling your burned hand under water will only throw you into physical chaos and could cause very serious damage that could have been prevented had you let yourself put your burned hand under cool water several times. If you don't the burn only gets worse, and the damage from the burn magnifies the less you take care of it. This is the same way it is with my needing several hugs. Not being able to do so is physically detrimental to me and physically and emotionally chaotic. It is too much for me to bear.

I have to be able to hug people I like and I have to be able to do it often. It is the only way I can handle it. I can't have it any other way.

There is actually a picture of a nurse hugging an elderly woman on page 25 of the Fundamentals of Nursing textbook in Figure 2-3. It says "providing nursing services in assisted living facilities promotes physical and psychosocial health" and this nurse is doing so by giving this lady a hug just as I am asking you to do for me.

> Fundamentals of Nursing, 7th Edition, page 25, Figure 2-3, Potter and Perry, Mosby Elsevier, 2009

"Effects of Sensory Deprivation include increased need for socialization, and altered mechanisms of attention in Cognitive areas."

> Fundamentals of Nursing, 7th Edition, page 1345, Potter and Perry, Mosby Elsevier, 2009

"As a nurse, you need to meet the needs of clients with existing sensory alterations and recognize clients most at risk for developing sensory problems."

> Fundamentals of Nursing, 7th Edition, page 1343, Potter and Perry, Mosby Elsevier, 2009

"Nursing care needs to provide mental and physical stimulation, particularly for a young child."

> Fundamentals of Nursing, 7th Edition, page 1250, Potter and Perry, Mosby Elsevier, 2009

"Nurses can use touch and eye contact to enhance a client's self-esteem."

> Fundamentals of Nursing, 7th Edition, page 417, Potter and Perry, Mosby Elsevier, 2009

"Touch is a primal need, as necessary as food, growth, or shelter. Think of touch as a nutrient transmitted through the skin and "skin hunger" as a form of malnutrition that has reached epidemic proportions in the United States, especially among older adults (Fontaine, 2005).

> Fundamentals of Nursing, 7th Edition, page 784, Potter and Perry, Mosby Elsevier, 2009

"Older adults need touch as much as or more than any other age-group. However, skin hunger or poverty of touch is often acute among older adults. It is an unfortunate coincidence that older adults often have fewer family members or friends to touch them at a time when simple touch could be an enhanced form of communication when other senses are reduced (Dossey and others, 2005)."

> Fundamentals of Nursing, 7th Edition, Box 36-5, page 784, Potter and Perry, Mosby Elsevier, 2009

"Simple touch helps older adult clients feel more connected to and accepted by those around them and to their environment. Touch enhances self-esteem and sense of worth. A nurse who reacts adversely to the skin changes of older people often finds it difficult to touch an older client. The nurse's reluctance then communicates a negative message to the older adult (Dossey and others, 2005)."

> Fundamentals of Nursing, 7th Edition, Box 36-5, page 784, Potter and Perry, Mosby Elsevier, 2009

"A holistic nursing approach to care of older adults also includes the caregivers, who often experience poor health or have neglected their own health, encounter their own psychological issues as they relate to the care giving experience, feel the effects of multiple stressors, or feel spiritual distress. (Eliopoulos, 2004)."

> Fundamentals of Nursing, 7th Edition, Box 36-5, page 784, Potter and Perry, Mosby Elsevier, 2009

"The ability to attend to the learning process depends on physical comfort and anxiety levels and the presence of environmental distractions. The nurse ensures that clients, families, and communities receive information needed to promote, restore, and maintain optimal health. In today's fast-paced technical environments, nurses are required more than ever to bring the sense of caring and human connection to their clients (see Chapter 8). Touch is one of the nurse's most potent forms of communication. Nurses are privileged to experience more of this 'intimate' form of personal contact than almost any other professional. Touch conveys many messages, such as affection, emotional support, encouragement, tenderness, and personal attention. Comfort touch, such as holding a hand, is especially important for vulnerable clients who are experiencing severe illness with its accompanying physical and emotional losses. In older persons, touch increases a sense of safety, increases self-confidence, and decreases anxiety (Geleeson and Timmons, 2004).

Fundamentals of Nursing, 7th Edition, pages 353,354, Potter and Perry, Mosby Elsevier, 2009

"Research has found that in children having a lumbar puncture, a medical procedure, a nurse's soothing nonessential touch decreased anxiety and lowered the child's distress (Bannorshdall and others, 2004). Students may initially find giving intimate care stressful, especially when caring for clients of the opposite gender (Seed 1995)."

Fundamentals of Nursing, 7th Edition, pages 353,354, Potter and Perry, Mosby Elsevier, 2009

Students learn to cope with intimate contact by changing their perception of the situation. Since much of what nurses do involves touching, you need to learn to be sensitive to others' reactions to touch and use it wisely. Touch should be as gentle or as firm as needed and delivered in a comforting, nonthreatening manner."

Fundamentals of Nursing, 7th Edition, pages 353,354, Potter and Perry, Mosby Elsevier, 2009

"The nurse uses touch to communicate." (Figure 24-02), page 354
> Fundamentals of Nursing, 7th Edition, page 354, Figure 24-2, Potter and Perry, Mosby Elsevier, 2009

"The nurse establishes, directs, and takes responsibility for the interaction, and the client's needs take priority over the nurses' needs. The nurse's nonjudgmental acceptance of the client is an important characteristic of the relationship. Acceptance conveys a willingness to hear a message or to acknowledge feelings. It does not mean you always agree with the other person or approve of the client's decisions or actions. A helping relationship between nurses and client does not just happen – you create it with care, skill, and trust."
> Fundamentals of Nursing, 7th Edition, page 346, Potter and Perry, Mosby Elsevier, 2009

"Therapeutic interactions increase feelings of personal control by helping the person feel secure, informed, and valued. Creating a therapeutic environment depends on your ability to communicate, to comfort, and to help clients meet their needs."
> Fundamentals of Nursing, 7th Edition, page 346, Potter and Perry, Mosby Elsevier, 2009

"Health is a "state of complete physical, mental, and social well-being, not merely the absence of disease or infirmity. Health is a state of being that people define in relation to their own values, personality, and lifestyle. Each person has a personal concept of health. Health and illness must be defined in terms of the individual."
> Fundamentals of Nursing, 7th Edition, page 748, Potter and Perry, Mosby Elsevier, 2009

"The nurse's presence helps to calm anxiety and fear related to stressful situations. Giving reassurance and thorough explanations about a procedure, "remaining at the client's side", and coaching the client through the experience all convey a presence that is invaluable to the client's well being."
> Fundamentals of Nursing, 7th Edition, page 784, Box 36-5, Potter and Perry, Mosby Elsevier, 2009

I noted these two things on a chart of Watson's 10 Carative Factors, one carative factor was "forming a human – altruistic value system. An example in practice for this is to "use loving kindness to extend yourself." You use self-disclosure appropriately to "promote a therapeutic alliance with your client." Another example in practice in promoting and expressing positive and negative feelings is to "support and accept your clients' feelings. In connecting with your clients you show a willingness to take risks in what you share with one another." It also says another carative factor is "providing a supportive, protective and/or corrective mental, physical, societal, and spiritual environment." An example of this would be to "create a healing environment at all levels, physical and nonphysical. This promotes wholeness, beauty, "comfort", dignity, and peace."

> Fundamentals of Nursing, 7th Edition, page 98, Table 8-1, Potter and Perry, Mosby Elsevier, 2009

On page 131, Figure 10-3 a nurse holds a patient's hand and puts her other hand just below her shoulder on her arm as she talks to her.

> Fundamentals of Nursing, 7th Edition, page 131, Figure 10-3, Potter and Perry, Mosby Elsevier, 2009

A nurse on page 129 in Figure 10-2, possibly at a nursing home is observing family interactions when they put a puzzle together actually leans over and helps them put some of the pieces of the puzzle together. She assists in understanding family functioning by doing this.

> Fundamentals of Nursing, 7th Edition, page 129, Figure 10-2, Potter and Perry, Mosby Elsevier, 2009

This is an example of just how relational a nurse is supposed to be. Some nurses may just stand off to the side and think, "I'm just going to mind my own business while this family puts a puzzle together" but this nurse interacts with her patients and tries to make them feel at home and helps to entertain them.

> Fundamentals of Nursing, 7th Edition, page 129, Figure 10-2, Potter and Perry, Mosby Elsevier, 2009

Try to learn to be more involved with your patients and interact with them and do everything you can to keep them happy and comfort them affectionately when they need you to. Don't just act standoffish, be a good nurse and show motherly compassion to all those in your care and put their minds at ease when they come to you.

The Fundamentals of Nursing Book says this about Emotional Comfort on page 347, Box 24-5. "Recently hospitalized clients described emotional comfort as a pleasant positive feeling and state of relaxation that resulted from therapeutic interactions. Clients described emotional discomfort as unpleasant negative feelings and tension. Personal control over the situation contributed to emotional comfort. Therapeutic interactions helped the client achieve control and were associated with emotional comfort. Clients perceived a positive link between emotional comfort and recovery"

> Fundamentals of Nursing, 7th Edition, page 347, Box 24-5, Potter and Perry, Mosby Elsevier, 2009

It goes on to say the following about Application to Nursing Practice: "Clients perceive a connection between the mind and body. Increased emotional comfort increases physical comfort and enhances recovery. Nurse-clients therapeutic interactions improve the client's emotional and physical comfort. Using therapeutic communication to increase the client's perceived control of the situation and the environment increases comfort." (Williams AM, Irurita VF: Emotional comfort: the patient's perspective of a therapeutic context, Int J Nurse Study 43 (4); 405; 2006.

> Fundamentals of Nursing, 7th Edition, page 347, Box 24-5, Potter and Perry, Mosby Elsevier, 2009

In the Fundamentals of Nursing book on page 131 you will see in Figure 10-3 that a female nurse is holding a patient's hand and puts her other hand just below her shoulder on her arm as she talks to her.

> Fundamentals of Nursing, 7th Edition, page 131, Figure 10-3, Potter and Perry, Mosby Elsevier, 2009

In Figure 25-3 on page 377 a female nurse puts her arm on a male patient's back when they walk them down the hall.

> Fundamentals of Nursing, 7th Edition, page 377, Figure 25-3, Potter and Perry, Mosby Elsevier, 2009

In Figure 27-4 on page 417 a female nurse touches a male patient on the arm with her hand. The statement under this picture says, "Nurses can use touch and eye contact to enhance a client's self esteem."

> Fundamentals of Nursing, 7th Edition, page 417, Figure 27-4, Potter and Perry, Mosby Elsevier, 2009

On page 482 in Figure 30-7 a female nurse puts her arm around their colleague during time of loss to support them. This is a nurse comforting a nurse. The same should go for nurses toward patients in their loss as well.

> Fundamentals of Nursing, 7th Edition, page 482, Figure 30-7, Potter and Perry, Mosby Elsevier, 2009

In the Reader's Digest: "Your Body Your Health, The Heart" there is a friendly female nurse on page 128 that puts one hand under a male patient's shoulder while checking his heart with a stethoscope with the other hand.

On page 131 of "Your Body, Your Health, The Heart" there is a female nurse putting her arms around the arm of a male patient to help him walk forward. She seems to be guiding him along so he won't fall.

> Reader's Digest: "Your Body Your Health – The Heart", page 128, Reader's Digest Association, London, 2002

This nurse may have not necessarily done this to comfort this patient, but at least she was showing compassion by being willing to put her arms around his arm to hold him up instead of standing back and saying, "I'm a professional. I can't do that. I'm not touching anybody. You'll just to have to hold on to a guard rail and walk on your own."

I've never heard anyone make that particular statement in this area of care before, but, they have said similar things to me in similar circumstances. And this is what it feels like when nurses act like they think they are so professional to the point they refuse to touch you or let you touch them. The more they act like this, the more you begin to get the feeling one of them might actually do something like this if they wanted to get out of touching you. Nurses are supposed to comfort their patients and any nurse that thinks they are not supposed to comfort their patients is wrong. Any nurse that thinks this way needs to go back and reread their own books. A lot of the information I got to write in the second half of this book came out of a college textbook of nursing, and it's not old either, it's a 2009 version. I didn't get it out of a 1970s book like I did some of my earlier encyclopedia references. I also need to remind you though that not all of my encyclopedia references were that old. Some of them were from 1985, some were from 2006, some were from 2014, and a few were even from 2016. It's still the same story. You're the nurse and you are supposed to comfort your patients. Even the college text book I found on nursing says this several times. It even comes out and tells you how to comfort your patients in several instances and actually tells you to use "touch therapy" to comfort your patients. In other words, this book is also telling you to comfort your patients with the hand holds and the head rubs and some of this other stuff I'm asking you to do. And, the Nursing Career CD I found with a book for nurses seeking careers in nursing it showed nurses rubbing the heads of patients, stroking their face, and holding their hands several times. And, they weren't old people or children either, they were my age. I'm 47 years old and these people appeared to be in their 30's, 40's, and 50's. Seeing that, it is not just limited to seniors and children, and it shouldn't be. Comfort from nurses should be for all stages of life, and one of the recourses I quoted said so as well. Comfort should not be delegated to end of life care as they said and people of all ages should be comforted by their nurses. Believe it or not, even though some nurses have been picky about comforting me I've run into the past couple of years, there are some that I've run into over the past 10 years that are more than happy to meet my needs. Many of them even call me sweetie, or honey, or bud, or buddy.

I've ran into some people in the public that will complain and say, "I just can't stand it when they do that. I'm not their honey. And, I'm not their sweetheart." And, you know what I have to say to them, "What's wrong with you? I like it when my nurses call me honey and sweetheart, and buddy. I think it's sweet, and I feel like they think I am special to them when they do this for me. I think it's great." They all give me lots of hugs that are like this and they will rub my head to calm me down and hold my hand through a needle stick. The problem was that only certain departments would go along with this in my old hospital and I needed nurses in all departments to be this way instead of acting all pompous and stoic and standoffish refusing to comfort me because they thought they were some kind of a professional that worked for a business somewhere like it was a firm or something, when in fact they were a nurse, not my business associate. I didn't come to do business with them, I came to be "cared for" by them because they are supposed to "take care of me" because they are my "caretakers" and nurses are your caretakers, not your business associates.

In a doctor's office or hospital setting, and especially the hospital setting, the nurses are basically supposed to take the place of your mother and treat you as if you were one of their own kids and comfort you in the same manner as they would their own child or baby, because they are "taking care of you" as a mother would "take care" of a child, and you are their patient, and they are now supposed to take on the role of the parent, and supply all the comfort you need in the way you need them to comfort you and not the way they decide they want to comfort you. Nursing a patient is not about the nurse, but the patient. It's not about the nurse's rights, it's the patients. And when you read your own college books as I did mine when I went to school, you will see when you read it that it tells you in your own school book, "It's not about the nurse's rights. It's about the patient's rights." It's the patient that matters and you need to be willing to resort to doing whatever they need you to do for them like a mother would a child. Nurse means to nurture, and any nurse that is not willing to comfort their patients like they would their own child or baby should not be a nurse and should find a different profession to work in.

"Caring facilitates healing and improves client satisfaction with nursing care. However, does the instructional process influence human caring? Do nurse educators present instructional methods that improve students' caring practices? Undergraduate nursing students received a 15 week educational module on nursing as human caring. The purpose of the module was to improve students' understanding of caring practices and to thus make them more caring practitioners. Researchers interviewed the students before and after completing the module to understand the effect of this module on their caring practices. For example, they asked students about factors that facilitated and impeded their caring practices. The students reported an increased self-awareness in regard to (1) connecting in relationships with self and others, (2) finding purpose and meaning in life, and (3) clarifying values."

> Fundamentals of Nursing, 7th Edition, page 98, Box 8-2, Perry and Potter, Mosby Elsevier, 2009

"Several students spoke of becoming more tolerant of others, recognizing persons' uniqueness and appreciating their perspectives. By recognizing themselves as caring persons, the students gained meaning in their lives. Many were able to relate a great deal of satisfaction in recognizing that they were caring persons and how nursing allowed them to express that. Students worked through the emotional issues and practical constraints, which allowed them to grow spiritually and connect with clients at a deeper level. Finally, students also expressed and enhanced appreciation of what they valued."

> Fundamentals of Nursing, 7th Edition, page 98, Box 8-2, Perry and Potter, Mosby Elsevier, 2009

"Application to Nursing Practice in enhancing caring is increasing knowledge and understanding of caring helps nurses begin to understand a client's world and to change their approach to nursing care. The use of caring in nursing practice encourages a more therapeutic approach to nursing care. As nurses use caring, they get to know their clients and therefore better meet their needs."

> Fundamentals of Nursing, 7th Edition, page 98, Box 8-2, Potter and Perry, Elsevier, 2009

"The caring model involves a closeness, commitment, and involvement in the nurse-client relationship."
> Fundamentals of Nursing, 7th Edition, page 98, Box 8-2, Potter and Perry, Elsevier, 2009

"An advocate is a person who speaks or acts for another person. As the resources and personnel involved in health service increase, there is an increasing need for someone who will take responsibility for explaining, interpreting, defending and protecting patients' rights. The primary orientation of nursing is toward human well-being. The nurse is most concerned with the ways a patient is experiencing what is happening to him. This may not always be the primary concern of other health care workers. A nurse may need to speak for a patient at times when he cannot speak for himself. Patient advocacy goes beyond direct patient care. It includes involvement in decision-making procedures concerning health services at local, state and national levels. Whenever health-related issues are being debated, nurses should be represented to ensure that a humanitarian approach to total patient care is maintained."
> Basic Nursing: A Psychophysiologic Approach, Sorenson, Luckman, 1979, W. B. Saunders Company, page 59

Nurses that know the "special needs" of a patient, particularly one who is disabled like me, should advocate for the patient to other nurses and doctors at other doctor's offices and hospitals to assure the patient's special needs are met. I have a really good family doctor who is a female Advanced Nurse Practitioner who does this for me and things go really well when she does because this is what I need and she makes sure my needs are met by everyone. I really want to thank her and tell her I appreciate her for this greatly. Thank you.

As, I said, I think everything is finally set now, but I certainly hope so. I am very happy with the new doctors I have and appreciate their willingness to meet my childlike needs. And, thank you to my new doctor, or technically, my new nurse practitioner who understands my needs and is willing to meet them. I really like my new family doctor, or technically, my nurse practitioner.
She is the friendliest, nicest nurse I've ever met. I hope she likes this book and I hope she continues to do everything she can to meet my needs and see that others meet my needs too. She tops every doctor I've ever had. She has the personality I always wanted in a doctor. She actually looks and acts exactly like a friend of ours at a bible camp we know. You can't find a better doctor than that when they act like one of your favorite friends. She is the sweetest, most wonderful doctor I ever met, except she's a nurse practitioner. I thought we'd never find a doctor like her. She is very nice. I'm really happy with her. It's very rare to find a doctor that nice. I'm glad we have her for our nurse practitioner instead of a regular family doctor. I am very pleased with her. Thank you for being willing to meet my needs and actually meet them. You're the most wonderful doctor, technically, nurse practitioner I've ever met. Thanks for everything.

Your friend,
Brian Gene Evans.

Dear Nurses,

Please note my needs when you take care of me. I appear to be
normal but I am actually autistic and have childlike needs. I need a
lot of affection from cheery acting, chipper female nurses with
motherly personalities who are caring and compassionate and
willing to comfort me the way I ask them to comfort me. I have a
sensory issue in my right ear that can only be relieved by putting
my right ear on the cheek of the people I like, I call doing this a
hug. So, I need to be able to do this with my nurses as well to
bring me comfort, especially in medical situations, and I need to do
it even worse when I'm scared. A cheery acting female nurse also
needs to rub the top of my head and hold my hand to comfort me
through an IV stick, blood test or shot, while another cheery acting
female nurse does the stick. They also need to do this for me if I
have a biopsy awake or have to be stuck with or cut with any other
sharp instruments. It is really important I have these met. Those
who have done this for me in the past did really well with me. I
have a fear of needles and oversensitivity to pain. A shot and a
blood test feel like being stuck with a steak knife. An IV feels like
being stabbed with a butcher knife. A catheter feels like a sword
being run through me. I need to be able to put
Lidocaine/Prilocaine 2.5% cream on the site of the stick because of
this. I need to be knocked out for all invasive procedures, as well
as any catheter or tube insertions. I also need all the radiology
techs and anesthesiologists and everybody that deals with me
needs to be cheery, chipper acting females only and I need to be
able to put my right ear on their cheek too because of my sensory
issue. Male doctors, nurses, and techs tortured me as a child so I
am scared of men. The serious trended female nurses also tortured
me in childhood and adulthood so I am scared of them too. Please
give me chipper acting, cheery female nurses to work with me
only.

Dear Nurses,

For those of you who are unable to catch what all of my needs are on the letter you just saw who need to see them in list form, here is my list of needs again. Please meet all these needs on this list. Not doing so traumatizes me, so it's very important you meet these.

- Need All Chipper Acting, Cheerful Female Nurses Only
- No Male Nurses, Therapists, Techs, Radiologists, or Anesthesiologists
- No Serious Trended Female Nurses, Therapists, Techs, Radiologists, or Anesthesiologists
- Need Hugs from All My Nurses (A Hug to Me is Putting my Right Ear on Your Cheek)
- Need a Chipper Acting, Cheerful Female Nurse to Rub my Head to Calm me Down and Hold my Hand While Another Chipper Acting Female Nurse does the IV, Blood Test, or Shot
- They Also Need To Do This For Me If Any Biopsies are taken awake, or any Blades, Or Scalpels, or Other Sharp Instruments Are Used On Me Awake
- I Need to Be Able to Put on Lidocaine/Prilocaine 2.5% Cream on Site of Stick
  One Hour Before A Needle Stick of Any Kind
- Need to Be Knocked Out For Any Catheter Insertions or Tube Insertions
  (Heart or Urinary Catheter Insertions)
* Need to Be Able to Write Doctors/Nurses About Any Medical Conditions/Symptoms   I Have or Any Emotional Needs I Need Met
* Need All Medical Professionals Dealing With Me to Be Informed of the Needs
  On this List and Be Willing to Meet Them

You meet this list and we are good to go. I still need to hug everyone I see so don't just limit it to one or two people that specifically work with me.

I need to be able to hug everybody I see when I go for a test in the Radiology Department for example, or the Pre-Op Department for example. Being able to do this helps me to be able to feel safe in my environment and comfortable with my nurses with the reassurance that anyone who does any other test on me in the same department will always be the same way with me as well as the ones that work with me, but do still only give me the chipper acting female nurses only to work with me because they are the nurses I am comfortable with. Plus, I have a sensory issue in my right ear that can only be relieved by being able to place my right ear on the cheek of all the people I like, including nurses. Not only that, but there are some tests that are so difficult for me to handle you may need extra assistance at times as well, so it is also better that everybody be prepared to give me a hug so I can feel at ease with everyone and know I will be taken care of in the way I need cared for with the comfort I need to receive from them in the way I need to receive it from them and not by what they decide but by how I tell them they need to comfort me, by giving me hugs, let me press my right ear on their cheek, and rub my head to calm me down and hold my hand through needle sticks. I need chipper acting cheery female nurses only to work with me.

The chipper acting cheery female nurses are the most compassionate people that do better at comforting me and making me feel at ease than anyone else. Male nurses and serious trended nurses tortured me as a child. Serious trended female nurses also tortured me as an adult. I need the chipper acting female nurses only to work with me that have cheery motherly personalities and comfort me the way I state I need comforted and I will be good to go. I am autistic and have childlike needs and need to be comforted in the way I ask to be comforted because this is the only thing that works for me. Please see to it that this is done for me, and we're set to go. Thank you.

Your friend,

Brian Gene Evans

To Read more about my life as a person with autism, be sure to read Autism Undiagnosed Part I – What Happened? , Autism Undiagnosed Part II- Will I Always Be An Outcast? And Autism Undiagnosed Part III- Joys and Sorrows of Living with Adult Autism, a three part series by my wife, Bertha Marie Evans.

Thank you. I hope you had a nice read and I hope this book gave you a better understanding of the needs I have that I need met by all my nurses in the medical field.

Also available are…

Victory: What Everybody Wants by Bertha Marie Evans

How to Have a Happy Marriage: Getting Past the Differences by Bertha Marie Evans

To schedule Bertha Marie to talk to your church group or organization, contact her at (870) 416-1030 or (870) 416-8912.

She is an expert in adult autism, addiction, and abuse not only by study but by real life experience.

New Books Available by Brian Evans (or) Brian Gene Evans

"Big City Hospitals Don't Like Cowards"

"Mainstreaming a Disabled Person into the Normal World is a Big Mistake"

"What Language Therapy Really Entails"

"Compassion for Disabled Peers in College is Needed"

www.ingramcontent.com/pod-product-compliance
Lightning Source LLC
Chambersburg PA
CBHW070253190526
45169CB00001B/397